erase your waist

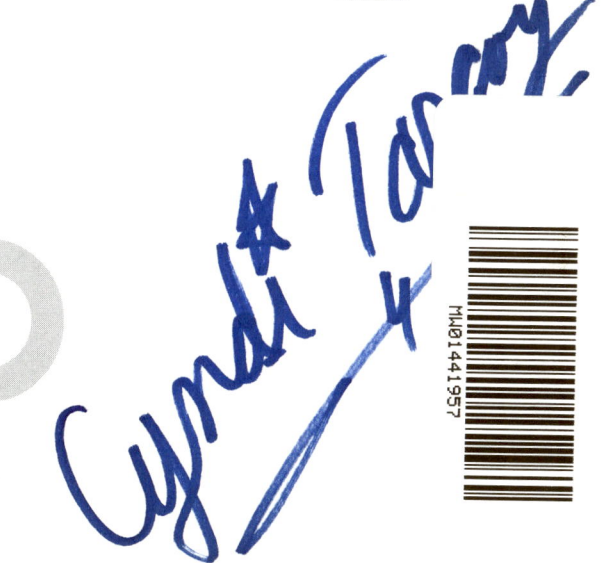

erase your waist

in minutes a day

cyndi targosz

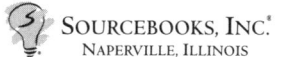
SOURCEBOOKS, INC.
NAPERVILLE, ILLINOIS

Copyright © 2005 Starglow Productions, Inc.
Cover and internal design © 2005 by Sourcebooks, Inc.
Cover photographs © Punchstock
Internal photographs courtesy of Kelsey Edwards Photography
Sourcebooks and the colophon are registered trademarks of Sourcebooks, Inc.

All rights reserved. No part of this book may be reproduced in any form or by any electronic or mechanical means including information storage and retrieval systems—except in the case of brief quotations embodied in critical articles or reviews—without permission in writing from its publisher, Sourcebooks, Inc.

This publication is designed to provide accurate and authoritative information in regard to the subject matter covered. It is sold with the understanding that the publisher is not engaged in rendering legal, accounting, or other professional service. If legal advice or other expert assistance is required, the services of a competent professional person should be sought.—From a Declaration of Principles Jointly Adopted by a Committee of the American Bar Association and a Committee of Publishers and Associations

This book is not intended as a substitute for medical advice from a qualified physician. The intent of this book is to provide accurate general information in regard to the subject matter covered. If medical advice or other expert help is needed, the services of an appropriate medical professional should be sought.

Published by Sourcebooks, Inc.
P.O. Box 4410, Naperville, Illinois 60567-4410
(630) 961-3900
FAX: (630) 961-2168
www.sourcebooks.com

ISBN 1-4022-0261-X

Library of Congress Cataloging-in-Publication Data

Targosz, Cynthia.
  Erase your waist / by Cyndi Targosz.
     p. cm.
  ISBN 1-4022-0261-X (alk. paper)
 1. Physical fitness for women. 2. Abdomen—Muscles. 3. Exercise for women. 4. Women—Nutrition. 5. Weight loss. I. Title.
RA778.T357 2004
613.7'1'082—dc22
                                          2004003517

Printed and bound in the United States of America
         VP   10 9 8 7 6 5 4 3 2 1

This book is dedicated to my beloved late father, Stanley J. Targosz, Sr. He taught me to live life to the fullest and enjoy each moment. He would always say, "This is really living!"

Advisory Note

Not all exercises are suitable for everyone and this or any exercise program may result in injury. To reduce the risk of injury, never force or strain in performing the exercises. The exercises are designed for persons who are in good health and are physically fit. Please consult with your medical advisor before beginning this or any other exercise program.

The creator, author, publisher, producers, participants, exhibitors, and distributors of this program disclaim any liability or loss in connection with the exercises or advice contained in this program.

Acknowledgments

There have been so many wonderful people who have supported me throughout my life and on this project. I wish to extend my sincere gratitude and thanks to all of them.

To my beautiful family including my parents, two brothers, five sisters, and their spouses, my nieces, nephews, aunts, uncles, and cousins. I love you all.

To my dear friends and associates who have always believed in me and what I stand for:

Dr. Jeffrey Anshel, Lila Baron, Marty Bernstein, Debra and David Budge, William Felber, Erik Feuchuk, Mike Fisher, Trudi and Mauri Friedman, Jim Gates, Teri Gianneti-Sergeant, Bill Gladstone, Shirley Goodman, Michael Goodman, Demetria Katsihtis, Paul Kirby, Mark Levin, Bernie and Estelle Meadows, Leslie McClure, Linda and Paul Ottosi, Gary Owens, Mark and Lyn Proffer, Sandy Pollock, Augustus Raney, Lynda Razo, Gary Ross, Jim Spencer, Kitty Spencer, Sr. Seraphine, Anastasia Taylor, Gina Traficant, Elaine Traskos, Kimberly Valentini, Sonya VanSickle, Beth Young, Kelsey Edwards Photography, my editor Deborah Werksman at Sourcebooks, and all the others too numerous to name who have contributed so much to me along the way.

Table of Contents

Introduction viii

Chapter 1: Tummy Talk 1
  Who This Program Is For 1
  How It Works 2
  Belly Image 2
  Genetics 3
  Tummy Touch Time 5
  Belly Bloat 6
  Spot Reduction 6
  Body Composition 7
  Basic Abs and Lower-Back Anatomy 8
  Charge It! 9
  Workout Choices 10
  Equipment Needed 10
  Tummy Terms 11
  Body Mass Index Table 14

Chapter 2: Body Type Basics 15
  Ectomorph 16
  Endomorph 18
  Mesomorph 20
  Body Type Blends 21
  Additional Fashion Tips 22

Chapter 3: Warm-Up 24
  Aerobic Warm-Up 24
  Aerobic Warm-Up Exercises 25
  Warm-Up Stretches 27

Chapter 4: Workout 34
  The Abdominal Section 35
  The Lower Back Section 50

Chapter 5: Cool-Down 58
Relax 59
Exercises and Equipment 59

Chapter 6: Posture and Breathing 69
Poor Posture Slump 69
Posture Check 70
Instant Non-Surgical Tummy Tuck 71
Diaphragmatic Breathing 71
Breathing Check Exercises 72
Posture Check Exercises 75

Chapter 7: Nutrient Knowledge 80
Water......................................81
Vitamins....................................82
Minerals....................................86
Protein.....................................87
Carbohydrates................................88
Fat 89

Chapter 8: Nutritionally Yours 91
To Diet or Not 91
Pyramid Power and Beyond 92
All Calories Are Not Created Equal 96
Serving Size..................................97
Alcohol Consumption 98
Food Journal..................................99
Food Labels 99

A *Not*-So-Final Note from the Author 102
About the Author 104

Introduction

My Dear Reader,

You did it! You just picked up the key to erasing your waist. This is not the first abdominal workout book that has ever been on the market. Nor will it be the last. It is, however, the one that is in your hands right now. The one that will work for you if you let it. Cling to it. Open it up and devour the information. Not only will I show you how to develop your best abs, but I will take you on a fascinating journey that goes beyond fitness. Welcome to the world deep within your womb. Use this key to open the door to a new discovery of self. It's all in your hands.

Love,
Cyndi

chapter 1

Tummy Talk

Your tummy is talking to you. She's hungry. The poor thing wants to be healthy and in shape, but doesn't know what to do. You have tried everything—diets, exercise, and more. She just won't listen. You look at her in scorn every day and quickly cover her up as best as you can. Sound familiar? It's about time that you became friends with your belly—she is part of the core of your whole being. You really can learn to love yourself. Let me share with you my secrets for how to Erase Your Waist. Fill up on this information and your tummy will growl no more.

Who This Program Is For
- She is bombarded by images in the media of beautiful, slim abs.
- She longs to have her own personal best-sculpted abs.
- She may have had a baby and wants to lose the excess fat.
- She is contemplating liposuction but is afraid of negative results or can't afford it.
- She may have had liposuction and wants to maintain strong, healthy abs.
- She wants to learn about her body type so that she can set realistic ab goals.
- She wants to know which clothes work best for her body type.
- She wants nutrition information simply explained.
- She is young.
- She is mature.
- She is you!

How It Works

Erase Your Waist is a very individualized program. I've designed it so that you can achieve your personal best abs. It begins with an explanation of genetic variances. Once you understand your body type, I will help you set realistic goals and even give you some great fashion tips to help you enhance your God-given traits. I then show you how to do a complete abs warm-up, workout, and cool-down that will tone your tummy, trim your waistline, and strengthen your lower back. There are also some great posture and breathing exercises that contribute to a strong core, or middle area. You will love the fact that good posture and breathing can instantly take off the appearance of up to ten pounds. On top of that, there are pages of sound nutritional advice. You will learn that enjoying food is a good thing. It's a matter of making healthy, educated choices. Finally, throughout the book, I encourage you to build strength not only in your muscles, but also in the power of the beauty you have within.

When done consistently, this program really works. *Erase Your Waist* is not a complete exercise regimen, but it is a *necessary* addition to your regular workout. It's also a great place to start if you are new to exercise or haven't worked out in awhile. Your regular program should include all-over body muscular endurance, strength, flexibility, and cardiovascular fitness. Since your core, or middle area, is critical for health and good looks, *Erase Your Waist* is a must! Do the complete program three to four times a week on alternate days to get results. No matter what your age or tummy size, the time to tone up is now!

Belly Image

When you hear the word "belly," what image does it conjure up? Many women automatically say, "Yuck!" I find this response disturbing—the belly is a beautiful part of the female anatomy. Certainly, I encourage you to try to eliminate excess fat for health reasons. However, not everyone can have

a six-pack. Although rock-hard abs can look phenomenal, so can a tummy that is firm, toned, and strong with a little bit of a belly. As women, we need to appreciate our personal best differences. I say "as women" because I believe that when it comes to the tummy, women are harder on themselves than men are on women. Most men actually prefer a pretty, toned belly on a woman. My mission is to help you achieve your personal best abs, and also to help you learn to love them. Let's discuss genetics, and then I'll explain an uplifting exercise I call Tummy Touch Time. Use this information to inspire a positive belly image.

Genetics

There are several different genetic reasons why some people develop more pronounced abs than others. It would take several medical books to explain it in detail. For our purposes, we will look at how muscle fiber makeup and childbearing affects ab development.

Muscle Fiber Types

Understanding the skeletal muscle fibers will help you appreciate why your ab results are so personal and individual. Muscle fiber consists of the following two types:

1. Slow Twitch Fibers (slow muscle contraction)—These fibers work best with aerobic activities (e.g., running). Aerobic means "with oxygen."
2. Fast Twitch Fibers (fast muscle contraction)—These fibers do not have the aerobic capabilities of slow twitch fibers. Think of fibers used in weightlifting, for example.

Most people have a mix of slow and fast twitch fibers that are distributed fairly evenly throughout their bodies. For world-class athletes, the distribution is usually not as balanced. A top professional long-distance runner would probably use 60 to 90 percent slow twitch muscle fibers.

A world-class power weightlifter would use around 60 to 90 percent fast twitch muscle fibers.

Understanding the composition of muscle fiber types in your body will help you set personally realistic goals for yourself. This doesn't have to be complicated. For example, if you do best with aerobic activities, you probably have a higher percentage of slow twitch fibers. If strength training is your forte, you probably have a higher percentage of fast twitch fibers. There can even be variations between your different muscle groups, such as more strength in the legs than in the arms. This is all very normal.

Fast and slow twitch fibers are found in both men and women. There is no physiological difference in terms of fiber distribution. In my own experience, I have found that men tend to be naturally stronger (fast twitch) in their upper body than women, while women have relatively stronger legs. Research shows that although you cannot change a genetic muscle fiber type, you can change the way it responds. That explains why if your abs have a high concentration of fast twitch fibers, a fabulous six-pack is realistic for you. If you have a higher concentration of slow twitch fibers, you can achieve a beautiful strong, firm, and toned tummy. Therefore, whether you have a larger percentage of slow twitch fibers or a larger percentage of fast twitch fibers in your abs, you can still get realistic positive results. Genetically, if your ab muscles are mostly slow twitch fibers, it may take a little longer to experience any physical change, but it will happen. Be patient and don't compare yourself to anyone else.

The message to you is to accept your unique genetic makeup. Know that whether you have a large amount of fast twitch or slow twitch fibers, you will be able to get a significant improvement in the appearance of your tummy.

Childbearing

A woman's body is built to have children. During childbirth, the entire hip, abdominal, and pelvic area expands. In general,

women either carry their baby primarily in the front so that there is more expansion through the abs, or they carry the baby farther back so that there is more expansion in the hips. If your body is built to carry a child more toward the front, it only makes sense that it might take a little longer to lose the front ab fat after childbirth. Don't let this discourage you. Whether you carry your baby forward or back, your body is going through natural changes. After childbirth, use the *Erase Your Waist* program to help you shape up.

Tummy Touch Time

Now that you are aware of some of the genetic factors that contribute to your waist potential, let's look at you. Whether you are trimming off twenty extra tummy pounds or honing in on a six-pack, if you don't have a positive belly image, your abs routine will never be successful. How do you achieve that positive belly image, you ask? It's Tummy Touch Time!

Tummy Touch Time is an intimate exercise I've developed specifically for women. It's a perfect complement to the *Erase Your Waist* program. The underlying premise is that if you don't love yourself right now, in this moment in time, you will never have a positive belly image. Learning to love yourself, and I mean *really* love yourself inside and out, will help you move mountains in every area of your life.

You can begin Tummy Touch Time in the privacy of your home when you are alone. Take off all your clothes and stand naked in front of your mirror. That's right—naked! Place both hands on your bare belly and watch the beauty of the movement as you slowly inhale and exhale. Feel the heat radiate from your womb. Notice the softness and texture as you touch your stomach. Caress your curves and love every ounce of your flesh. Look in the mirror again, naked—face the truth. My program will help you Erase Your Waist to your best potential, but it is up to you to discover you!

Belly Bloat

It's not unusual for a menstrual cycle to affect a woman's disposition. Even thin women have so-called "fat days." Have you ever known intellectually that you hadn't gained any weight, but emotionally you felt heavier? You can blame the hormone progesterone for that feeling. About a week before your period, your body begins to produce increased amounts of progesterone. It's the progesterone that retains the fluid. Its purpose is to prepare the egg for fertilization. This fluid hangs out around the stomach, creating that bloated feeling. Once the body realizes that there is no pregnancy, the progesterone reverts back to its normal level, the excess fluid is excreted, and your tummy feels like you again.

My hope is that through the *Erase Your Waist* program, you will develop a better appreciation for the natural cycles in your life. The changes that take place in your body are part of being a woman. Self-acceptance and understanding of this normal biological process will make coping with the symptoms easier.

Tip: If during PMS you have a hot date, it is exceptionally important to eat healthy foods and avoid those that cause bloating and gas. Foods that I find helpful during PMS are:

- Citrus fruits
- Whole grains
- Water
- Fish
- Green leafy vegetables

Spot Reduction

In order to get maximum results out of the *Erase Your Waist* program, you must understand that you cannot spot reduce. I don't care how many sit-ups or crunches that you do—the fat will not just melt away in one body part area. When you lose weight, it comes off your entire body. What you *can* do is firm and tone up the underlying muscles of your belly as you lose all-over body fat. That's exciting!

To Erase Your Waist, you must do *all* of the following:

1. **Burn fat**—Do something that will use oxygen to get your heart rate up. Chapter 3 has an excellent selection of aerobic activities. Select one of them or another activity that you enjoy. Do it for at least thirty minutes, three times a week for a full cardiovascular workout. Do not skip this component or you will never see the tone-up results. They will be covered by fat.
2. **Tone up**—Do the exercises I've prescribed for you in the warm-up, workout, and cool-down chapters. They will firm your abs to your personal best shape.
3. **Breathe properly**—Explained in chapter 6.
4. **Maintain good posture**—Explained in chapter 6.
5. **Eat a balanced diet**—Explained in chapters 7 and 8.

Body Composition

Body composition is the percentage of body fat that you have relative to your muscle mass. In many ways, your body composition is far more important than any number on a scale. A scale doesn't take into account the weight of your bones and muscles compared to your body fat.

A famous test for body fat is the pinch test. You know, the one where you are supposed to squeeze your love handles with your fingers. If you can grab more than an inch of fat from your waist, some experts say you need to lose weight. Please! Do you really have to pinch yourself to know that you might be getting a little fat? I personally think the pinch test is counterproductive and a waste of time. It's a negative process.

One of the most accurate ways to measure body fat is with a system called hydrostatic testing. This method requires a special tank that measures body fat after an individual is completely immersed in water. Since most people are more likely to own a Jacuzzi, bathtub, or shower stall than a hydrostatic tank, I thought I would offer another method of measurement.

The Body Mass Index (BMI) is not a perfect measurement, but it will provide a guideline for you. It indicates body composition by using your weight relative to your height. For your convenience, I've included a Body Mass Index table at the end of this chapter (page 14). The top numbers represent approximate body fat percentages. In general, anything over 25 percent body fat for women and over 30 percent body fat for men is considered obese.

Basic Abs and Lower-Back Anatomy

As you work at sculpting your abs, it's useful to understand the anatomy of your midsection. This will help to create a visual aid when you are doing the exercises. The term *abdominals* is the name for the muscle group commonly called the abs. I've also included a description of the lower back muscle group. The abs and the lower back work together to create a balanced core area.

Rectus Abdominus

This is a long vertical muscle that makes up your front midsection. It runs from the lower chest to the pubic bone. The *rectus abdominus* is a major component of your core area. Keeping it strong will help your whole body work more efficiently. It is a key component of body stability. It also is used to help you bend. It helps you flex your rib cage toward your hips or your hips toward your rib cage.

Most people refer to the top and bottom half of the muscle as the upper and lower abs. It is actually one long, flat muscle. The upper part is divided into three paired segments, giving it the common name six-pack. The bottom half, which falls below your belly button, is divided into two segments. If you add those segments to the six-pack, it's actually more accurate to call the rectus abdominus an eight-pack muscle. Since most women want to tone both the upper and lower abs, I've included exercises in the *Erase Your Waist* program that will stimulate muscle fibers in both areas.

Oblique Abdominus
This muscle group runs at an angle along the sides of your torso from the lower rib cage to the pubic area. It is actually two muscles: the internal and external obliques. You have a pair on each side of your waist.

The external and internal obliques help you to rotate at the waist. They also assist the rectus abdominus for bending movements and contribute to core stability. Each pair of obliques helps you to bend at the side.

Transverse Abdominus
This is a thin horizontal muscle that cuts across your abdomen. It is important for core stability, helps with breathing, and holds your internal organs in place.

Erector Spinae
This is a powerful muscle group in your lower back. It should never be neglected in the *Erase Your Waist* program. The *erector spinae* runs along the lower spine. It helps with maintaining good posture, takes your torso out of a bent position, helps to maintain stability, and assists the obliques during any waist rotation.

By strengthening the erector spinae, all of your body movements will work more efficiently. A strong lower back will help you avoid back injuries. It also helps the ab exercises to be more effective.

Charge It!
Credit cards are a large part of our lives, because so many of us love to shop! I knew that concept would capture your attention, and that's why I'm using it. Just as you shop for a pair of shoes or a dress to make you look and feel your best, it's also up to you to shop for healthy lifestyle information. That makes it your responsibility to take *charge* of your own body. The *Erase Your Waist* program is chock full of information that will take you to a new level of health, beauty, and

fitness. What you do with this knowledge is in your control. I say, take charge!

Workout Choices

The wonderful thing about this program is that it offers a lot of flexibility to fit your lifestyle. You have choices!

1. You can do the complete warm-up, workout, and cool-down three to four times a week on alternate days. Include the posture and breathing exercises in chapter 6.
2. You can turn the aerobic warm-up in chapter 3 into a complete cardiovascular workout by increasing the duration of your selected activity to thirty minutes or more. Gradually increase intensity at the start of your activity (warm up) and gradually decrease the intensity at the end of the activity (cool down). Do this three times a week.
3. Posture and breathing exercises in chapter 6 should be done at least twice a week.
4. The warm-up and cool-down can be done as often as you like. Many women enjoy the relaxing effect that these exercises have and the increased flexibility that they offer. They are a treat! When planning your workout week, enjoy them all as a healthy bonus—but for *Erase Your Waist* results, you *must* do the exercises in chapter 4 and those for posture and breathing in chapter 6.

Equipment Needed

Below is a list of all the equipment needed in the *Erase Your Waist* program. When you get to a specific workout section, I'll let you know which of these items is necessary at the time.

- Fitness Mat, Towel, or Rug
- Barbell
- Chair or Sofa
- Flat Workout Bench—A flat stool would also be perfect.

- Hand-Held Weights—It's best to start out with light weights, such as two to five pounds. If that is too heavy or you have never exercised before, try the movement with no weights until you have mastered the technique. Soup cans are an excellent inexpensive alternative.
- Stability Ball—These are very popular now in a number of fitness programs. You can pick one up at any sporting goods store for about thirty dollars. However, you always have the option of doing the same move on the floor without the ball. Be aware that doing so will decrease the level of difficulty.

Tummy Terms

Following are some terms that you will see throughout this book. I hope this helps you to increase your knowledge base. Perhaps you can come to terms with your own tummy.

Abdominal muscles (Abs)—This is the technical term for the stomach muscles.

Aerobic—A workout that uses oxygen, e.g., running.

Amino acids—The building blocks of proteins.

Biceps—A muscle that has two heads of origin on the front of the upper arm. This helps to bend the forearm.

Body composition—The percentage of body fat that you have relative to your muscle mass.

Calorie—A unit of energy.

Carbohydrates—These essential nutrients provide energy for the body. Examples are simple sugars and complex carbohydrates.

Cardiovascular—The use of the heart to move large muscle groups over a sustained period of time.

Core strength—Working the abdominal and lower-back muscles.

Diaphragm—A muscular membrane separating the thoracic cavity from the abdominal cavity.

Diaphragmatic breathing—The emphasis is on using the diaphragm to breathe rather than the chest cavity.

Ectomorph—A body type with a long, lean build.

Elongate the spine—To extend the spine to a greater length for better postural alignment (i.e., stand straight.)

Endomorph—A body type with a round build.

Fast twitch fiber—A muscle fiber that contracts at a fast speed. Most often associated with activities that are anaerobic or don't need oxygen, e.g., weightlifting.

Fat—This essential nutrient insulates the body and provides energy.

Fat-soluble—Nutrients that cannot be dissolved in water, so they are stored in fat.

Fetal position—The position of the fetus in the womb.

Glucose—A sugar that occurs in the body.

Hamstring muscles—These muscles make up the back of your leg. They are responsible for any leg pulling action (e.g., pull your heel up to the back of your thigh.)

Hypoglycemia—Low blood sugar.

Liposuction—Removing fat through surgery.

Mesomorph—A body type with a strong, muscular build.

Metabolism rate—The rate in which the body breaks down food into energy.

Monounsaturated fat—A type of unsaturated fat that has one hydrogen atom, e.g., olive oil.

NLEA (Nutrition Labeling and Education Act of 1990)—A law requiring most foods to have a visible nutrient label.

Pilates—This workout was originally designed to rehabilitate injured soldiers during World War I. When its founder, Josef Pilates, brought his techniques to the U.S., they were done by dancers to lengthen the muscles to improve flexibility and strength. Pilates is done on a machine that is composed of pulleys and cables, or on a mat. Movements are slow and controlled and include deep breathing.

Polyunsaturated fat—A type of unsaturated fat that has more than one hydrogen atom, e.g., corn oil.

Progesterone—a hormone that prepares the body for fertilization.

Protein—This essential nutrient builds and repairs body tissues.

Quadriceps—The largest group of muscles in your body. They are made up of four individual muscles in the front of your leg. They help you to extend the lower leg.

Repetitions—How many times you do an exercise (e.g., ten wall pushes).

Resistance training—When an opposite force such as a weight or gravity is used to strengthen your muscles.

Saturated fat—A type of fatty acid that has the maximum amount of hydrogen atoms.

Set—A group of repetitions.

Slow twitch fiber—A muscle fiber that contracts at a slow speed. Most often associated with aerobic activities.

Stability ball—A ball used to improve balance and tone muscles.

Thoracic breathing—Using the chest cavity to breathe rather than the diaphragm. This is not recommended for these exercises.

Trans fats—polyunsaturated oils that are saturated with hydrogen atoms.

Triceps—The muscles in the back of your arm. They are used to extend the forearm to push things away, including yourself, such as in a pushup.

Urologist—A doctor who diagnoses changes in the anatomy of the patient through the study of the urine and genitourinary tract.

Vertebrae—The bones of the spine.

Water-soluble—Dissolves in water.

Yoga—A form of exercise founded in India. It combines postures (stretches) with breath control and inward reflection.

Body Mass Index (BMI)

	19	20	21	22	23	24	25	26	27	28	29	30	35	40
Height (inches)							Weight (pounds)							
58	91	95	100	105	110	115	119	124	129	134	138	143	167	191
59	94	99	104	109	114	119	124	128	133	138	143	148	173	198
60	97	102	107	112	118	123	128	133	138	143	148	153	179	204
61	100	106	111	116	121	127	132	137	143	148	153	158	185	211
62	104	109	115	120	125	131	136	142	147	153	158	164	191	218
63	107	113	118	124	130	135	141	146	152	158	163	169	197	225
64	110	116	122	128	134	140	145	151	157	163	169	174	203	233
65	114	120	126	132	138	144	150	156	162	168	174	180	210	240
66	117	124	130	136	142	148	155	161	167	173	179	185	216	247
67	121	127	134	140	147	153	159	166	172	178	185	191	223	255
68	125	131	138	144	151	158	164	171	177	184	190	197	230	263
69	128	135	142	149	155	162	169	176	182	189	196	203	237	270
70	132	139	146	153	160	167	174	181	188	195	202	209	243	278
71	136	143	150	157	165	172	179	186	193	200	207	215	250	286
72	140	147	155	162	169	177	184	191	199	206	213	221	258	294
73	144	151	159	166	174	182	189	197	204	212	219	227	265	303
74	148	155	163	171	179	187	194	202	210	218	225	233	272	311
75	152	160	168	176	184	192	200	208	216	224	232	240	279	319
76	156	164	172	180	189	197	205	213	221	230	238	246	287	328

chapter
2
Body Type Basics

This chapter begins with the premise that nobody is perfect—and I do mean nobody! As you progress in the *Erase Your Waist* program, you *will* be able to look in the mirror and say, "Damn, I look good!" To get to a point where you can exude that kind of confidence, you need to understand that there is no such thing as perfection, and accept whatever body type you were born with.

In all of my experience as a professional in the health and beauty business, there is one thing that has remained constant. Women are rarely satisfied with their looks. I'm not just talking solely about the average woman on the street, but popular actresses and models who appear to have it all. The secret I share with you, as I have with many of my clients, is how to first accept your genetics and learn what you can do to flaunt the good stuff, and secondly, how to make those so-called "flaws" work for you.

Let's look at genetics. There are three basic body types: ectomorph, endomorph, and mesomorph. Most women fit primarily into one of these category but have characteristics from other categories as well. Appreciate your genetics; that's what makes each of us unique. Have fun learning which body type or blend of types you are. We'll discuss how that applies to your realistic goals.

We'll also have a little fashion fun. You will learn how to select clothes that enhance your specific body type. After all, a girl can never have enough basic body type tips to help her

take charge of her fitness, nutrition, and, of course, shopping plans. As you read, it is my hope that you will begin to see that beauty comes in more than one package size. Enjoy *your* special beauty.

Ectomorph

Attributes
If you are an ectomorph, you are basically tall, long, and lean. A classic ectomorph has long limbs—think runway model.

An ectomorph is often the envy of others because she can eat enthusiastically and not gain weight. Her delicate structure usually includes slim hips and pelvis. A typical ectomorph has very little fat and small muscle mass.

As an ectomorph, your small body fat percentage is one to be hailed. You can attribute that to a naturally faster metabolism rate. That just means you are able to burn off fat faster than other body types—even when you are sleeping.

When it comes to a workout, you excel in cardiovascular endurance activities. Your aerobic capacity and long limbs allow you to run free like a gazelle. Flexibility is another strong point for the ectomorph. That's a big plus considering that mobility will help you avoid injury in the later years of life.

Recommendations
Now that you've heard all the wonderful things about your fashion plate figure type, you probably think you are home free. I hate to have to tell you, but being healthy goes far beyond being thin. In fact, sometimes I'll hear famous actresses and models who are thin ectomorphs brag about the fact that they don't exercise and are able to eat anything they want. People think they are automatically healthy because they still look so great. Sure, the outside may appear beautiful, but here's a lesson for all women—being slim does not always mean that you're fit. Sometimes the reverse is true. If you don't exercise, watch what you eat,

(and follow the *Erase Your Waist* program), it is possible that your internal organs and body functions are out of shape. I suggest you look beyond skin deep. If you don't take care of yourself, you are prone to heart problems, high cholesterol, diabetes, and a number of other health issues. It's conceivable that your heavier friends are healthier and more fit than you.

If you are an ectomorph, I'm going to recommend that you take extra care to eat properly and stay active. Follow my nutrition advice in chapters 7 and 8. Be sure to do all-over muscle toning exercises, including the *Erase Your Waist* program. Lucky you! Since you probably have very little fat to begin with, you will be able to focus on toning up faster than other body types. Unfortunately, since your body responds better to aerobic activities, muscle sculpting can sometimes take a little longer. However, if you are consistent in your healthy food choices, your favorite aerobic activity and flexibility moves, and if you continue to tone up, your tummy will have the taut look you desire.

I've seen excessively thin women with poor muscle tone who actually have a higher percentage of body fat than muscle—dangerous for inner health. I've also seen ectomorph women who have totally let themselves go and don't even look like ectomorphs anymore. If you are an ectomorph or a blend with other types, face yourself from within. Take advantage of your genetic potential, and strive for your personal best.

Fashion Tips—Ectomorph
- Belts work great for you; they add curves.
- Pleated skirts and dresses will fill out your figure.
- Long, narrow jackets and tops will help you accentuate a tall, willowy look.
- Maintain good posture (see chapter 6). Ectomorphs can appear gawky if not standing proud.

Endomorph

Attributes

If you are an endomorph, you probably have been called curvy, voluptuous, and shapely. Great artists have captured the beauty of endomorph women in drawings, oil paintings, and sculptures. Have you ever experienced a magical museum visit where you saw radiant Renaissance and Rubenesque women brought to life on canvas? Their pounds of flesh flaunted femininity in each pose. I doubt these women dared to ask their significant other, "Do I look fat?" They were too confident in themselves. (Well, at least I imagine that they were.)

When experts use the term endomorph, they are simply describing the female shape as that of an hourglass. Many famous movie stars and models for men's magazines have capitalized on this fabulous form.

Unfortunately, endomorphs can also put on weight quite easily, particularly in the lower body—the abs, butt, hip, and thigh areas. Classic endomorphs have short limbs in proportion to the rest of their body. Their muscle tissue has a tendency to be on the soft side. Bone structure for the most part is that of a small or medium frame.

Recommendations

As an endomorph, you have the potential to walk into a room and cause jaws to drop—"Wow!" It may take a little more effort since your body type tends to carry excess fat, but you can do it. Do not, however, expect to achieve a model-thin body. This doesn't mean that you could never work as a high fashion model—I like to think that the industry is becoming more open to different body types. I also believe that if there is a will there is a way. However, accept the fact that your bone structure cannot be something that it is not. Why set unrealistic goals? Enjoy your particular body type. Learn to love your natural curves.

Start by checking out your body fat percentage on the BMI chart in chapter 1. Healthy food choices and regular exercise are a must for you. Strive to feel better about yourself inside and out. The *Erase Your Waist* program is a natural for you. As an endomorph, your extra weight is most likely to be in the stomach area. This goes beyond looks. Studies have shown that a heavy middle area can lead to a number of health problems such as stroke, heart disease, and high blood pressure, to name a few.

I suggest that you think seriously about doing an aerobic activity as a full cardiovascular workout at least three times a week. Check out some of the options in chapter 3. You may have to work a little harder in this area than others, but the rewards are worth it. A cardiovascular workout will give you an advantage when you progress through the *Erase Your Waist* workout. You will lose fat and tone your tummy in no time. Although you might not have much muscle definition at the start, your potential for strength is tremendous.

It's not uncommon for endomorphs to develop a hopeless, "woe is me" attitude. They want to blame their body weight strictly on genetics. Certainly, genetics does play a big part. However, I am saddened by women who use it as permission to give up. Love and respect your natural curvy self enough to quit being a victim of circumstances. Choose to live a healthy lifestyle.

Fashion Tips—Endomorph
- Dark colors and solids can be slimming.
- If you've managed to create prominent curves as a result of working out, pastel colors will work fine. Congratulations!
- If heavy in the middle, avoid "shortie" tops.
- If clothing is too loose, it can make you look heavier. Better to go for a tailored fit.
- Wear long jackets and tops to balance your middle area.
- Pencil skirts can be very sexy on you.
- Avoid any pants or shirts gathered at the waist. They will make you look heavier.

Mesomorph

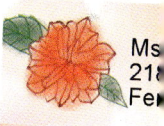

Attributes

If you are a mesomorph, you probably have the figure of a female athlete. Your muscles are quick to build definition and strength. Many marvel at your statuesque, rectangular, full-length shape. Because you have strong shoulders and well-developed chest muscles, your waist will often appear tinier than it really is. Mesomorphs generally have large, magnificent bones and muscles. It's much easier for you to sculpt your abs, hips, thighs, and other body parts than it is for the ectomorph and endomorph.

It is very in vogue to see women of your type taking center stage in movies, music videos, commercials, sports, etc. Strong, healthy muscles are the shape of today and the mesomorph woman can have them.

Recommendations

As a mesomorph, you have the potential to build beautiful strength and definition. People will gasp at how quickly you tone up. Unfortunately, all is not perfect. Mesomorphs can gain and store excess fat just as fast as they build muscles. This is especially true as they age and if they are not active. Are you an undercover mesomorph? It's time to emerge and reach your fullest potential. It's never too late to start. I'm going to recommend that you begin doing a full cardiovascular workout for a minimum of three days a week. Check out the options in chapter 3. It's important to find something you enjoy doing to ensure your success and it will aid in your exercise adherence. Review the nutrition information in chapters 7 and 8. It will help you balance your body composition with the food you consume.

Include strength and toning exercises. You may be able to get by with only two days of resistance training a week if you are building muscles at a fast pace. Be sure to continue with the *Erase Your Waist* workout. You have the potential to cut

. Stoltz
ɔdge Rd
N 56537

your abs into a shape that most women can only dream of. Remember to maintain good posture.

Fashion Tips—Mesomorph
- Your naturally strong shoulders do not need shoulder pads. You may have to remove them from certain apparel to maintain a balanced look.
- Avoid loose-fitting clothes. Opt for a tailored fit.
- Vertical lines will help give the illusion of being tall and thin.
- Avoid narrow-cut pants or jeans. They can make you look heavier.

Body Type Blends

By now you've read all of the different body type descriptions and have probably found characteristics within yourself that correspond to more than one type. The fact is that most people are a blend of body types. For example, you might have the strong muscles of a mesomorph, but the small bones of an ectomorph. That would make you a meso-ecto. You could also have the curvy waist of the endomorph paired with the strong, broad shoulders of the mesomorph. That would make you an endo-meso.

Decide which body type has your strongest features and work from there. Use the attribute information and recommendations that I give you for your particular body type or blend of types to help you understand your genetic makeup. Only then will you be able to set realistic goals. This will allow you to truly be able to see the beauty of your own individuality and appreciate the varied female forms of others. Use this information to help you take charge of your own body through the *Erase Your Waist* program.

Additional Fashion Tips

If Your Waist Is Long
- Avoid low-rise pants. They only make your torso look longer and your legs look short.
- Select pants and skirts that have a wide waistband.
- Short jackets are very flattering.
- Your belt should match your skirt or pants rather than your top to shorten the look of the torso.
- Thin vertical patterns on your skirt or pants will add the illusion of length.
- Horizontal lines on a blouse or jacket work fine.

If Your Waist Is Short
- Avoid gathered pants or skirts.
- Do not use horizontal patterns on your top. They will shorten the look of your torso.
- Low-rise and no waist pants or skirts look great on you.
- Your belt should match your top rather than your bottom to create the look of a longer torso.
- Tops that fall below your waist create the look of length.
- A short jacket will work, but only if you have a small waist and long, lean legs.

If You Have A Wide Waist
- Avoid A-line outfits.
- Wear soft shoulder pads for balance.
- Wear your coats, sweaters, and jackets open for a slimming look.
- Avoid belts if you can, since they accentuate the waist. If you choose a belt, make sure that it is thin.
- Body-hugging styles can work if they are straight and long to take the emphasis off the waistline.

If Your Tummy Bulges
- Avoid any thick fabric on your lower body.
- Metallic or shiny material will make a bulge more pronounced.
- Select longer tops.
- Horizontal collars will take the emphasis off the stomach.
- Soft shoulder pads will create balance.
- Pair longer tops and jackets with pencil skirts or narrow pants.
- Do not cover up in a completely baggy outfit in an effort to hide your bulge. This will make you look like a blimp. A tailored fit is much more attractive.

chapter
3

Warm-Up

Many fitness novices have the preconceived notion that a workout warm-up is for weenies. They are way wrong! Whether you are a seasoned athlete, a professional body builder, or an average woman trying to tone her tummy, the warm-up is a must in any fitness routine. The exercises in this chapter will increase your circulation and send blood and oxygen to your muscles.

Warmed-up muscles respond to a workout more efficiently and are less likely to get injured. That means faster results! I've selected this warm-up as a perfect compliment to the *Erase Your Waist* workout in chapter 4. It is divided into two sections: the aerobic warm-up followed by the warm-up stretch. They must be done in that order to achieve the safest and quickest ab response.

Aerobic Warm-up

To begin this program, you need to do something aerobic. An aerobic exercise is one that uses oxygen to get the blood circulation going. This will cause your body temperature to rise (hence the name "warm-up"). If done properly, your body temperature should increase by at least one or two degrees Fahrenheit.

This part of the program sets the pace and mood for the whole workout. Decide now. Are you with me or not? Because if you are, I am going to help you use that warmed-up body heat to make your beautiful belly the best it can be.

I always recommend choosing an aerobic warm-up activity that you genuinely like to do, so you are more apt to stick with it. You should do it for a minimum of five to ten minutes at the start of the *Erase Your Waist* program. To safely raise the heart rate, always start out slowly. At the conclusion of the aerobic warm-up, do not stop suddenly (which could cause unnecessary strain on the heart). Remember to keep breathing throughout the entire activity. After all, aerobic means using oxygen, so breathe! Always check your intensity level throughout any aerobic activity. You can easily monitor your intensity level by paying attention to the way you feel during the activity. If on a scale of one to ten, one means that you are feeling relaxed and ten means that you feel exhausted, you should strive to feel that you are at a level five. Another safe intensity level indicator is you ability to carry on a normal conversation while doing the aerobic activity.

An excellent add-on to this warm-up is to turn your aerobic activity into a full-blown cardiovascular workout. As I explained in chapter 1, you need to burn off calories and fat before you can see the results of your toned-up tummy. So why not increase the duration of your aerobic warm-up from five or ten minutes to thirty minutes or more? Always start and end at a safe, slow pace. Check your intensity level throughout. Feel good! Have fun!

Aerobic Warm-up Exercises

Following are a few aerobic warm-up options. You may know other activities that use oxygen that you would prefer to do. That's okay. In fact, it's not a bad idea to switch off for variety. Take charge!

1. Walk
2. Bicycle Ride
3. Shadow Box
4. Swim
5. Workout Step or Stairs

Walk
This aerobic warm-up activity is probably one of the simplest around, yet it is extremely beneficial. I personally walk quite frequently. Not only does it help physically, but the mental boost is phenomenal. (I probably wrote half this book in my mind during my walks.)

Tips: Maintain good posture throughout the activity. Stand tall. Use your heels to push off. Hold your arms at a 90-degree angle and pump them back and forth. Face forward. If you walk outside at night, wear light-colored clothing for safety.

Bicycle Ride
Whether you are on a stationary bike in your house or doing wheelies in your neighborhood, riding the bicycle for five to ten minutes minimum is a great aerobic warm-up.

Tips: Adjust your seat so that when your legs are in the down position there is a slight bend in the knee. It's okay to lean slightly forward on the handlebars, but keep your shoulders relaxed. The handlebars are there strictly for light support. When pedaling, avoid shifting knees out to the side. If you ride outside, wear protective gear.

Shadow Box
Who says you have to stand in a ring to get the aerobic benefits of boxing? Do it for a minimum of five to ten minutes and you are a champ in my book.

Tips: All you need is a mirror to watch yourself and a lot of spunk. Punch till your heart is content. Imagine beating down all your problems. They may not go away, but at least you will feel better. Silk boxing shorts are optional. Theme music from the movie Rocky *has been known to be helpful. You are #1!*

Swim

Perhaps you have access to a lake or other body of water. Lucky you! Enjoy the refreshing zip a nice swim will give you. A minimum of five to ten minutes gives you an aerobic warm-up with little impact on your joints.

Tips: For safety, never swim alone. Always rinse your hair after swimming and use a good deep conditioner. Chlorine and fresh and salt water can wreak havoc on a lasses tresses. If you can't swim, jumping and splashing in the water equates to an aerobic activity. Check your nearby sporting goods and pool stores for a selection of fun water toys such as paddle boards, beach balls, or water weights. (Floating cocktail cups and lounge chairs do not count as activity enhancers.)

Workout Step or Stairs

Almost everybody has access to stairs. If you don't, an inexpensive workout step will do just fine. A minimum of five to ten minutes of this up and down aerobic warm-up activity and you'll be ready to conquer the world.

Be sure to stand tall as you walk up and down. Try to avoid a tendency to lean too far forward from your waist, as that type of bending could injure your back.

Warm-Up Stretches

To Stretch or Not To Stretch?

Yes, that is the question, but don't think that it means I'm going to tell you to forget it. Although there are conflicting studies and opinions in the fitness world as to whether it is better to stretch before or after a workout, the key word is "or." It is pretty much unanimous that stretching is a necessary component of a workout. The debate is about when it is most beneficial.

For the purposes of this book, I have selected warm-up and cool-down stretches that are appropriate. The cool-down time

is lengthened for increased flexibility and relaxation. All the stretches are safe and effective. Since we are not running a marathon or using excessive weight, the when controversy is not as pertinent.

A word of caution—if you ever should choose to skip the warm-up stretch, remember never to skip the aerobic warm-up activity, and always do the cool-down in chapter 5.

Warm-up Stretches and Equipment

Below are some great warm-up stretches that I've specifically designed to prepare you for the *Erase Your Waist* workout.

1. Standing Abs
2. Twisting Torso
3. Barbell Twist
4. Pussycat
5. Hip Rotation

Here is a list of equipment needed for the warm-up stretches.

- Fitness Mat, Towel, or Rug
- Barbell—if you don't have one, a broomstick will also work
- Flat Workout Bench—a flat stool is another option

Standing Abs

This movement will really help you to get to know and feel your abs. It works the whole core area.

Start: Maintain good posture as you stand tall. Your feet should be hip-width apart. Raise your arms over your head with palms facing forward. Inhale. (See photo.)

Movement: Exhale slowly as you bring your arms down to your sides with palms facing inward. Simultaneously round your back, drop your chin to your chest, and contract or squeeze your abdominal muscles. Hold for 10 seconds. Go back to starting position. Repeat movement 10 times. (See photo.)

Tip: Make sure that you are squeezing your stomach muscles for the movement rather than using your hips or arms.

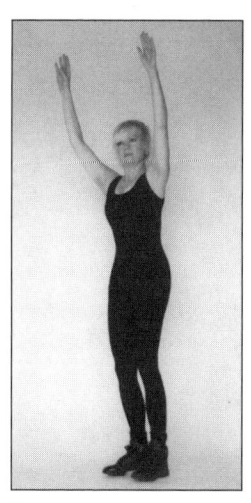

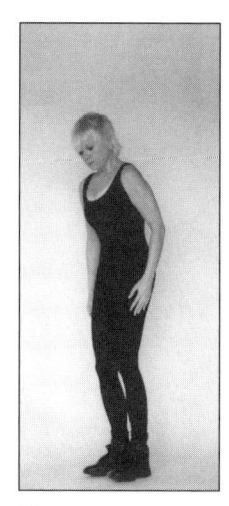

Start   Movement

Twisting Torso

This will warm up the joints of your neck, shoulder, and trunk.

   Start: Stand with your feet hip-width apart. Keep your body stable from the hips down.
Movement: Keeping your lower body still, twist your upper body while you look as far back behind you as possible and stretch your arms to the back. (See photo.) Hold for a moment and repeat on the other side. Do both sides 10 times each.

Tip: Avoid doing this move on thick carpet, which could make it more difficult to balance.

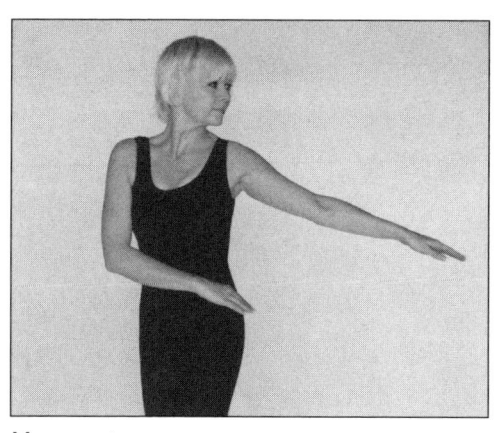

Movement

— 30 —

Barbell Twist

This is a fun warm-up stretch that will aid in whittling your waist.

Start: Sit on the end of a workout bench or on a stool. Your feet should be flat on the ground, but wide apart for balance. Place a barbell or a broomstick on top of your back and wrap your arms forward around it. (See photo.)

Movement: Keep the hips and lower body stable throughout this exercise. With a slow, continuous, and a controlled movement, twist your upper body to the far left and then to the far right. (See photo.) Do this 10 times to each side.

Tips: In the past, fitness experts had their clients twist quickly back and forth. We now know that a jerky movement is not good for the spine. Remember to keep the movement slow and controlled. Be sure the hips and lower body do not move.

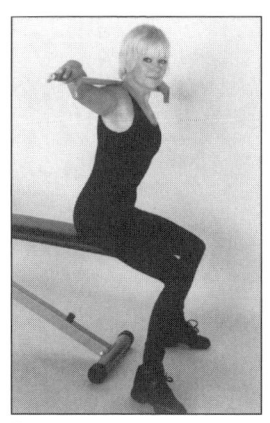

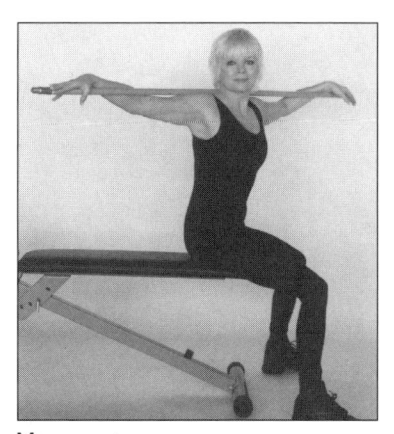

Start

Movement

Pussycat

This one's great for your abs and lower back. Purrrrfect!

Start: On your workout mat, get down on all fours. Keep your back flat. (See photo.) Inhale so that your tummy pouches out.

Movement: Exhale as you slowly pull your tummy in toward your back. Keep pushing your abs in as you round your back. (See photo.) You should feel good, like a sexy pussycat. Release and return to starting position. That is one repetition and should last 20 seconds. Repeat the move 3 times.

Option: You can make this move more advanced by contracting your abs from a modified push-up position. Your weight should be on your forearms and toes as you contract your abs.

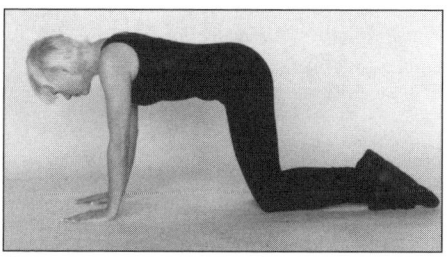

Start

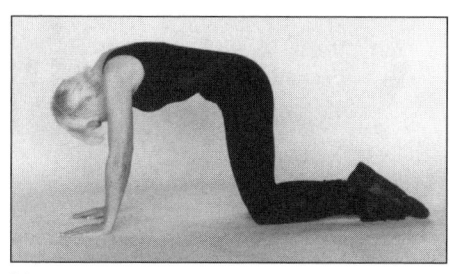

Movement

Hip Rotation

Great for lower back and torso.

Start: Lie on your back with arms out to the sides.
Movement: Bring your knees to your chest and slowly twist them from side to side. (See photo.) Repeat 10 times.

Tip: Be sure to keep the shoulders, arms, and upper body steady on the floor.

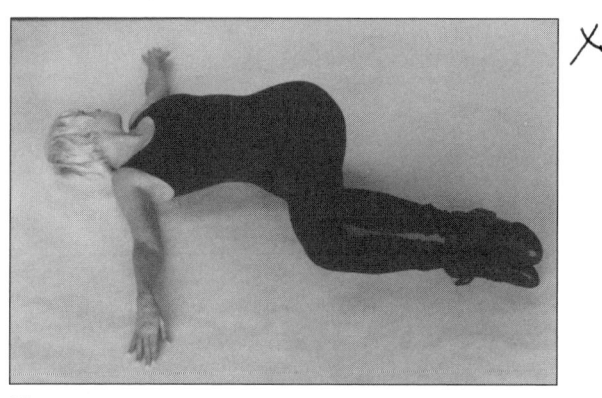

Movement

chapter 4

Workout

You are about to embark on the nucleus of the *Erase Your Waist* program. This chapter consists of abdominal and lower back exercises that will whip your midsection into shape. Whether you are an endomorph, ectomorph, mesomorph, or any combination thereof, doing these exercises will help you look and feel your personal best.

As you proceed through the program, you may start to dream up any number of excuses to avoid doing your abs routine. That's not unusual. Suddenly, even cleaning the house looks better than doing a workout. Even most fitness experts don't often say, "Gee, I can't wait to do my abs workout today." I tell you this not to discourage you but to help you acknowledge a normal human reaction. Only then will you be able to freely choose to do these exercises. Keep in mind that consistent completion of the movements will result in a slimmer, healthier torso. I personally look forward to doing these exercises because I know how good I'll feel when I'm finished. I choose to turn the workout challenge into a positive pleasure. You can use this knowledge as a form of self-empowerment. The discipline and motivation to crunch your core into shape will come from within yourself. You will be driven to personal excellence. If done consistently and properly, you will get results. You can do it!

I'm going to recommend that you do this routine at least three to four times a week on alternate days to get the best results. Do not let too many days of rest go by between

workouts. Proceed at your own level of difficulty. If you need to stop and rest during a set, that's okay! The good news is that they will get easier. It's far more important that you go at your own safe pace. Always do the warm-up in chapter 3 before your workout and always end with the cool-down in chapter 4. Have fun!

The Abdominal Section

Why The Abdominals?

When many women look in the mirror at their stomachs, they ask themselves the common question, "Do I look fat?" Merciless moments like that have sent masses of women into abs crunch madness. Perhaps that is what inspired you to pick up this book. If so, I'm glad. Because by doing the *Erase Your Waist* program consistently, you will see a great improvement in your outside appearance. A strong, taut tummy of personal best proportion will do wonders for the ego, but working the abs goes beyond visual appeal. These exercises will strengthen the muscles in your midsection core. Strong abdominals will help your whole body work much more efficiently. They affect everything from ease of arm and torso movement to your stability and posture. In fact, many women who suffer low back pain are actually experiencing the adverse effects of weak abs. The abs help you bend forward and backward and twist your torso. Do yourself a favor—fall in love with your new flat, fab abs, but embrace the strength you gain outside and in from doing the *Erase Your Waist* program.

Helpful Abs Workout Hints

Abs Order—When doing the abs exercises, the order in which you do them can make a difference in your results. Although I explained in chapter 1 that the rectus abdominus is really one long muscle, we will refer to it as the upper and lower abs. To make it easier for you to understand, the upper abdominals help out when you do exercises for the

obliques and lower abs. For that reason you shouldn't do upper-ab moves first because they would get tired and not be as strong as they should be for the other tummy moves. Saving the strongest muscles (upper abs) for last ensures the most efficient workout. Who has time to waste when working on the waist? I've arranged the *Erase Your Waist* exercises in the following order:

1. Obliques
2. Lower Abs
3. Upper Abs

- Breathe—When doing your abs routine, exhale when you contract the abs and inhale when you release them. Even if you get confused during a set, just breathe. The worst thing that you could do is to hold your breath.
- Range of Motion—When doing abdominal exercises, keep your range of motion at 45 degrees or less. In other words, when you move your torso up for a crunch or sit-up do not go beyond a 45-degree angle from the floor. If you do, you will be using your psoas or hip flexor muscles. Be aware this is a general rule. There are some advanced exercises where secondary muscles such as the hip flexors must be used to complete an ab move.
- Technique—Never employ poor technique in an effort to get extra crunches completed. When the abs fatigue, it's best to stop rather than use improper form.
- Speed—As a general rule, do these exercises with slow, controlled movements. For variety, feel free to vary the count. For example, when doing a crunch you could raise your torso up for a count of two and then lower it for a count of four, or vice versa. This will stimulate your muscle fibers and keep you from getting bored.
- Waistline Tip—Working the oblique muscles can certainly whittle the waist. Many women choose to do side bends with a weight in each hand to achieve slim sides. That popular

move is not recommended unless you want to build a wider waist. It could make you look like you are a heavier woman than you really are. Instead, opt to do the oblique moves in this chapter. They work!
- No Neck Lifts—A common mistake is to lift the head and neck up instead of lifting from the abs. This does nothing to trim the tummy and is a literal pain in the neck. If you visualize an orange between your chin and your chest it will help you avoid a wobbly head.
- Back Alignment—When doing abdominal exercises, do not arch the back and do not flatten it. When you hold the abs in, keep a slight space between the small of your back and the floor.

The Abdominal Results

You are probably wondering when you will see results! I refuse to give you false promises. It takes discipline and determination. Take charge! Simply follow the systematic approach I've prepared for you in the *Erase Your Waist* program and a beautiful belly will follow. The honest answer is that you must first get rid of excess fat that is covering your abdominal muscles. This can be achieved by doing cardiovascular activities and following a sensible diet. At the same time, you need to do your ab-sculpting exercises. If you are not more than five pounds overweight, you will start to see a visual change in approximately four to eight weeks. In four months, you can expect a feminine, trim look to your midsection. Stick with the plan, and in a year you will have your personal best, healthiest, strongest, most gorgeous abs. The good news is that even if you are excessively overweight you will immediately feel a good soreness in your abs. Be aware of the strength that is occurring in your core. As you lose fat, your toned tummy will be more visible. Enjoy the pleasure of the process of change. Let it inspire you to push on.

Exercises and Equipment

Following is a list of the abdominal exercises I've specifically designed to target the appearance and health of your abdominal muscles.

1. Oblique Crunch
2. Crunch with Side Flexion
3. Weighted Oblique Reach
4. Hip Swing
5. Lower Ab Lift
6. Legs Up Lower Ab Lift
7. Leg Push
8. Pilates Pump
9. Crunch
10. Curl Up
11. Ball Curl Up

Minimal equipment is needed for this segment of the process:

- Fitness Mat, Towel, or Rug
- Chair or Sofa
- Hand-Held Weights—It's best to start out with light weights, such as two to five pounds. If you have never exercised before or if the weight is too heavy, try the movement with no weights until you master the technique. Soup cans are an excellent inexpensive alternative.
- Stability Ball—These are very popular now in a number of fitness programs. You can pick one up at any sporting goods store for about thirty dollars. However, you always have the option of doing the same move on the floor without the ball. Be aware that doing so will decrease the level of difficulty.

Oblique Crunch

This exercise works the obliques or side ab muscles. Visualize a trim waistline.

Start: Lie on your back with knees bent up and together. Let them drop to your right side so that they are stacked on top of each other. Place your hands behind your head. Elbows should be on the floor to start so that the chest is open and facing up. Shoulder blades should be on the floor as well. (See photo.)

Movement: Exhale as you raise your shoulder blades off the floor and contract your abs. (See photo.) Slowly lower yourself back down. Do 20 repetitions on each side.

Tip: Keep your chin raised. Do not let it droop to your chest.

Option: You can turn this into an advanced exercise by using a stability ball. Lie sideways on the ball with legs out straight. Push your feet into a wall for balance. Place your hands behind your ears. Lift your shoulders as you crunch sideways.

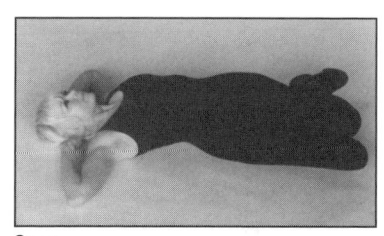

Start

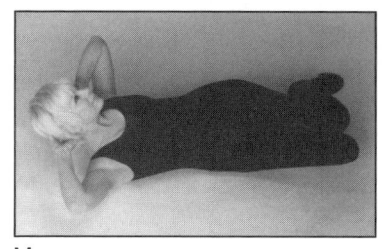

Movement

Crunch with Side Flexion

This is a great overall ab exercise. It especially emphasizes the obliques.

Start: Lie on your back with knees bent. Feet should be flat on the floor hip-width apart. Put your arms behind your head to open the chest. Keep your shoulder blades and arms on the floor. Inhale. (See photo.)

Movement: Exhale as you raise your upper body up. Keep the lower back pressed into the floor. Twist as you aim your left shoulder joint or armpit toward your right knee. The left armpit and right knee will not touch. This just gives you a direction to go to. (See photo.) Slowly return to start. Work up to 20 repetitions on each side.

Tip: Be sure to aim with your armpit and not your elbows to ensure that you are working the abs properly. It's a waste of energy to just flap your elbows back and forth. Try the move once using the elbows for direction and you will immediately notice that it is not as effective as reaching with your armpit.

Options: For greater difficulty, place the right knee over the left knee. For intermediate difficulty, place the right ankle on left knee. Remember to switch sides.

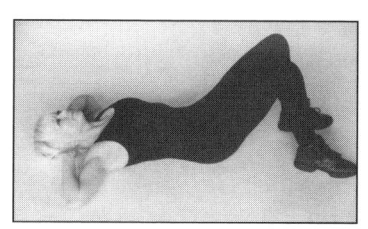

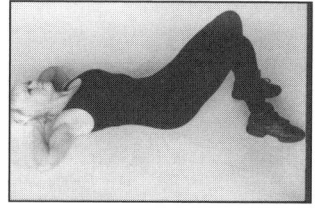

Start

Movement

Weighted Oblique Reach

Here's one for the upper abs and the obliques.

Start: Lie on your back with legs extended up towards the ceiling. Holding a two- to five-pound weight in each hand, extend your arms up as if to touch your toes. (See photo.)

Movement: Contract your abdominals as you reach up for your right baby toe. (See photo.) Slowly come down and immediately reach up for the left baby toe. That is one repetition. Work up to 10 repetitions.

Tip: Remember that how far up you lift your torso is not as important as maintaining good form.

Option: Rather than just twisting the abs toward the baby toes, feel free to include a set of ab crunches that lift straight up between your feet. That option will work primarily the upper abs.

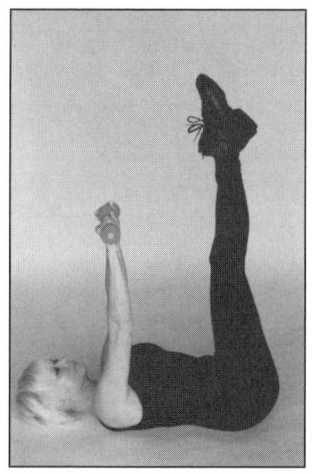

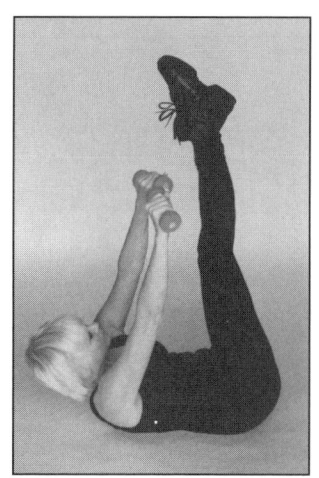

Start

Movement

Hip Swing

This works the obliques and the *rectus abdominus* with an emphasis on the lower back.

Start: Lie on your back with your knees bent and feet crossed. Place your hands behind your head with outstretched elbows. Bring your knees up to your chest with your crossed feet pointing up to the ceiling. Raise your upper torso off the floor, contracting your abdominals.

Movement: Stabilize your upper body as you lift your buns slightly off the floor. Gently swing your legs to the left. Contract your abdominals and aim to crunch your left hip toward the left shoulder. (See photo.) Return to start. Swing your legs to the right and repeat the movement. (See photo.) Work up to 20 repetitions, alternating each side.

Tips: Keep the upper torso still throughout the entire exercise. Be sure to exhale when you lift up to contract the abdominals. Concentrate on lifting your buns only slightly off the floor.

Options: For more of a challenge, let your buns swing from side to side without letting them rest on the floor. If the exercise is too difficult, simply perform the movement with your upper body on the floor and arms out to the sides.

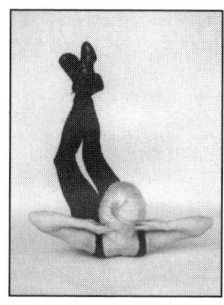

Movement   Movement

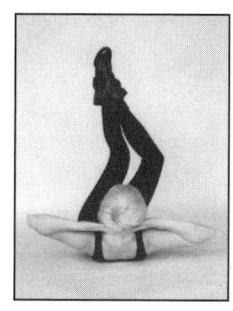

Lower Ab Lift

Flatten your paunch with this lower ab lift.

Start: Lie on your back with your arms at your sides. Bend your knees at a 90-degree angle so that your legs are raised off the floor with your knees pointing up to the ceiling and your lower legs parallel to the floor. Inhale. (See photo.)

Movement: Exhale and contract your abdominals as you lift your pelvis toward your rib cage. The tailbone should be slightly raised off the floor as you move your knees in the direction of your chin. Squeeze and hold your tummy tight for a second (see photo) and return to starting position. Work up to 20 repetitions.

Tip: Remember to use your tummy (abdominal) muscles to lift your pelvis rather than using your butt. This takes focus.

Option: For more of a challenge, do the same move on a stability ball. Lie on the ball on your back with your hips lower than your shoulders. You will need to hold on to a weighted object such as a chair for balance. Do the abs lift so that you curl your legs toward your chest.

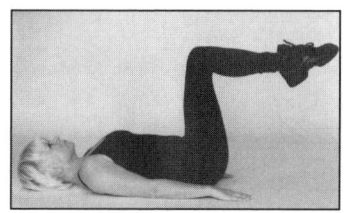

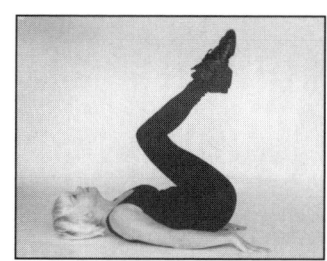

Start

Movement

Legs Up Lower Ab Lift

This is another great one for the lower abs.

Start: Lie on your back with your arms at your sides. Raise your legs toward the ceiling so that they are perpendicular to the floor. Inhale. (See photo.)

Movement: Exhale as you contract your stomach muscles to lift your hips slightly off the floor. (See photo.) Then lower your hips. Work up to 20 repetitions.

Tip: Focus on using your abdominals to lift your hips rather than using your buns to lift the hips. It is a subtle move that does not require you to lift your hips up high. If your hips are raised up too high, you are using your buns for the move. That is a completely different exercise.

Options: To increase the level of difficulty, place your hands behind your head during the exercise. If the exercise is too difficult, you can always do another set of lower ab lifts.

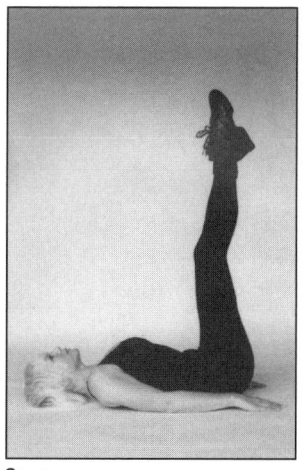

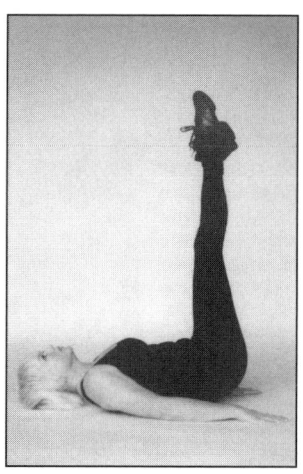

Start   Movement

Leg Push

This move works the lower abs.

Start: Sit on the floor with your arms behind you. Hands should be on the floor pointing forward. Bend your elbows so that you lean slightly back. Legs should be together and knees bent. Crunch your knees and chest together at the same time. (See photo.)

Movement: Inhale as you push your legs out at a 45-degree angle to the floor. (See photo.) Exhale as you return to knee and chest crunch position. Work up to 20 repetitions.

Tip: Repeat the movement in a slow and controlled rhythm. If you go too fast, you will be using the momentum to work with gravity, rather than working the abdominal muscles. That would be cheating yourself.

Option: To increase difficulty, hold your extended legs out for a count of four before returning to the knee and chest crunch position.

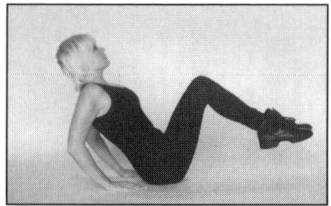

Start

Movement

Pilates Pump

This exercise, inspired by Pilates movements, works the entire abs area.

Start: Lie on your back with your arms at your sides. Lift your arms slightly off the floor. Bring your knees to your chest as you lift your head and shoulders off the floor. Now extend both legs up no lower than a 45-degree angle to the floor. Your lower back should maintain contact with the floor. (See photo.)

Movement: Keeping your arms straight, pump them quickly about an inch high up and down. Inhale for 5 quick pumps and exhale for 5 quick up and down pumps. Repeat for 10 repetitions of 5 inhalations and 5 exhalations, which adds up to 100 pumps. If you start to lose your form, stop the exercise. Finish by slowly elongating your body down to the floor—don't collapse.

Tips: Do not tense your neck. In fact, when you are first starting out you can hold it with one hand for support. Keep the abdominals contracted; try not to let them bulge out. Keep the spine in neutral alignment.

Options: To make the move easier, you can either bend your knees or raise your legs up higher than a 45-degree angle to the floor. To increase the difficulty, lower your legs below a 45-degree angle to the floor.

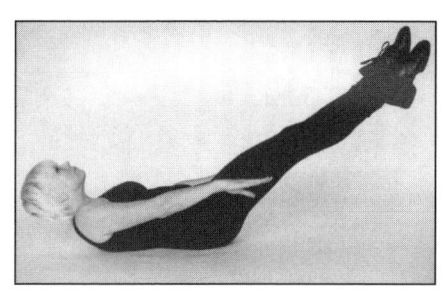

Movement

Crunch

This classic exercise works the upper abs.

Start: Lie on the floor with your knees bent and your feet flat on the floor. Fold your arms across your chest. Inhale. (See photo.)

Movement: Exhale as you contract your abs to lift your head and shoulders off the floor. (See photo.) Using a slow, controlled movement, return to start. Work up to 20 repetitions.

Tips: Make sure that you exhale during the contraction of this exercise. Remember to keep your chin up.

Options: To make the exercise easier, do it with the arms down at your sides. This shifts the center of gravity for a simpler position. If you would like more of a challenge, do the movement with your arms behind your head so that your hands are behind your ears. Do not interlock your fingers.

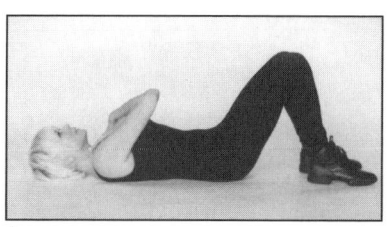

Start

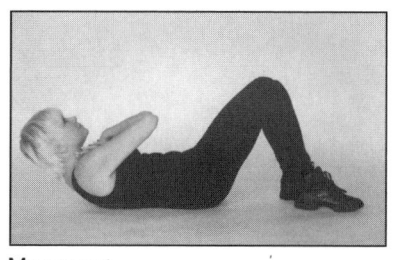

Movement

Curl Up

This exercise works the upper abs.

Start: Lie on your back with feet up on a chair. Cross your arms over your chest. (See photo.)

Movement: Exhale as you lift your upper torso toward the ceiling. (See photo.) Slowly return to start. Work up to 20 repetitions.

Tips: Be careful not to bring your chin to your chest. Focus on contracting your abs.

Options: Keep your arms out to the sides to make this move easier. For more of a challenge, place your arms behind your head during the exercise.

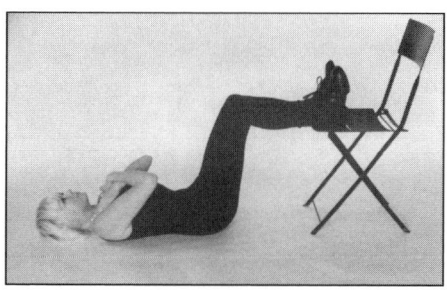

Start

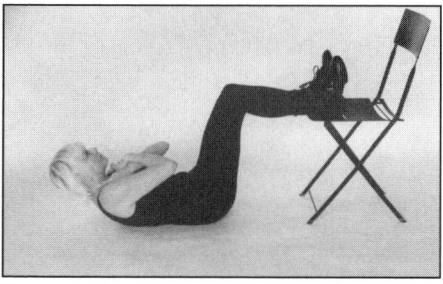

Movement

Ball Curl Up

This move works the *rectus abdominus* and the obliques. You will need the stability ball for this exercise. I love the way it forces the abs into a steady state of contraction. Very effective!

Start: Lie on top of the stability ball. Your feet should be placed flat on the floor in front of you, approximately hip-width apart. Put your hands behind your head with elbows out. Remember to keep a space between your chin and chest. Hold your abs tight so that your whole back, from the tailbone to your shoulders, is on the ball. Your arms and head should be held in place above the ball. (See photo.)

Movement: Exhale as you curl your upper torso off the ball. You will actually lift the head, neck, and shoulders. Pause a few seconds. (See photo.) Inhale as you return to starting position. Work up to 20 repetitions.

Tip: If you move slowly, it will help you to maintain balance.

Options: Part of the challenge in this exercise is that it requires you to maintain balance on the stability ball. If you find that the exercise is too difficult, you can do the same curl up on the floor. Once your abs are stronger, try using the ball again. To increase the level of difficulty, start with your head, neck, and shoulders placed back on the ball. Curl up from this lower position. Make sure that your abs are strong enough to attempt this advanced move so as not to injure the back.

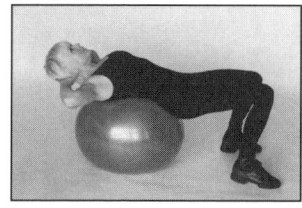

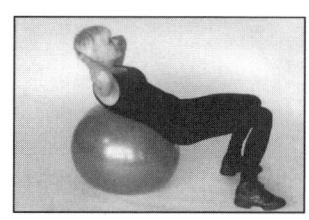

Start

Movement

The Lower Back Section

Why the Lower Back?

If you are even *thinking* about skipping this section, STOP right there! In order to achieve a streamlined, strong torso, the lower back region requires some undivided attention. As your personal trainer, I have to advise you of the many benefits you can gain by following my lower-back exercise prescription.

First of all, I'm a big proponent of balance. Everything in life—including your workout—needs balance if you wish to function in harmony. It is the beautiful synchronization of the right muscle movements with sharp mental focus that makes my program so successful. That is why every workout plan I design includes the opposite muscle group from the part of the body you are working. For example, if you work the front of the legs (quadriceps), you must work the back of the legs (hamstrings). If you work the front arms (biceps), you must work the back of the arms (triceps). Therefore, if you wish to tone your tummy, you must include the lower back in your workout for a balanced body and better results.

You may have heard that it's good to do ab exercises if you have lower-back pain. That is excellent advice, but only part of the equation. If you only train the abs and not the lower back, your muscles will be out of balance. When one of the muscle groups becomes stronger than the other, you are asking for trouble. It can throw your posture off, worsen your pain, and even create pains you've never had before.

Your lower-back muscles serve two functions. They help you bend your spine backwards and they stabilize your torso when you move another part of your body. It is the marriage of your abdominals and lower-back muscles that form your core of strength.

Another reason to work the lower back is because, in our society, we tend to spend a great deal of time sitting. Sitting puts a tremendous amount of pressure on the spine, much more than standing all day. Did you ever notice how your

back muscles ache after a day of work when you sit the whole time? With weak back muscles, there is a tendency to slouch, which puts even more stress on the back.

If all of that doesn't convince you of how critical lower-back strength is, consider your height. Working the lower-back muscles in conjunction with your abdominals will help you to stand tall. It will make you look leaner and more confident. If you ask me, that's enough to make any self-respecting babe get back into lower-back action.

Helpful Lower Back Hints

- Take Breaks—If you sit all day, take frequent standing breaks. This will help to relieve the pressure on your back.
- Check with Your Doctor—If you have chronic back pain, check with your doctor before beginning this or any other exercise program.
- If in Pain, Stop—The lower back is a sensitive area. While doing the exercises, you should feel a little stretch but not a sharp pain. If you are doing the exercises correctly and still feel pain, be sure to contact your health care provider.
- Don't Arch Too Far—While doing the exercises, be careful not to arch your back too far. If it is an extension move, it will help if you think about elongating your spine as much as possible.
- Don't Jerk—Slow controlled movements are the key to successful lower-back exercises. If you do quick, jerky movements, you may do more harm than good.

The Lower-Back Results Are In

Everybody wants quick results. Usually muscles in the back develop at a little bit slower pace than other parts of the body. Genetics, of course, does play a part in the rate of results. Generally, you can expect a positive change in six to eight weeks. You will immediately become more aware of your lower-back strength. This will aid in improved posture. The additional benefit is that lower-back strength can aid in

speeding up the results in your ab workout. Girl—you are on your way!

Exercises and Equipment

Following is a list of lower-back exercises that will compliment your ab workout for a prettier midsection. These will strengthen the lower back and aid in improving posture.

1. Dead Lift with Bent Knee
2. Pelvic Tilt
3. Bird Dog
4. Stability Ball Extension
5. Hang Straight

Equipment needed:
- Fitness Mat, Rug, or Towel
- Stability Ball

Dead Lift with Bent Knee

This is a great exercise that strengthens the lower back.

Start: Stand tall with feet shoulder-width apart.
Movement: Keeping your back straight, flex your hips and bend your knees until you reach down just below the knees. (See photo.) Push off your legs and use your lower back to return to starting position. Work up to 15 repetitions.

Tip: Be sure to keep your head up throughout the exercise.

Option: For more of a challenge, hold on to a light weight throughout the exercise. As your lower back gets stronger, you can increase the amount of resistance.

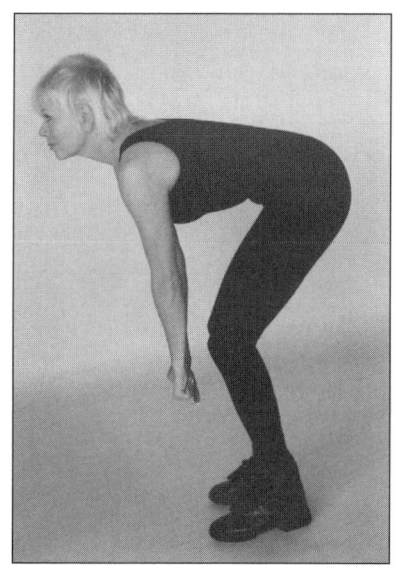

Movement

Pelvic Tilt

This tiny but effective movement gets you to concentrate on lower-back stability. It also includes the abdominals and hamstrings.

Start: Lie on your back with knees bent. Your feet should be flat on the floor about hip-width apart. Put your arms behind your head. Press your back down and contract your abdominals. (See photo.)

Movement: Press your back into the floor as you lift your butt and tilt your hips ever so slightly. Do not lift higher than an inch or two. Pause and hold this position for a few seconds. (See photo.) Slowly return to start. Work up to 20 repetitions.

Tips: Do not lift your head, neck, or shoulders; keep them relaxed. Do keep your lower back pressed into the floor throughout the entire exercise. Do not arch your back.

Option: To simplify this movement, try performing the exercise with your heels on top of a chair or sofa. Keep your knees bent at a right angle and your upper legs perpendicular to the floor.

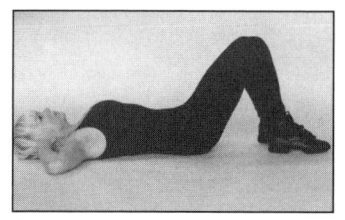

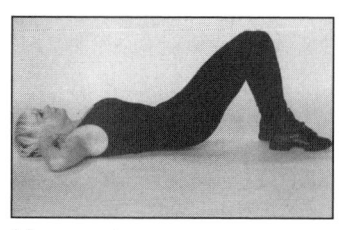

Start

Movement

Bird Dog

This classic extension exercise is a winner. It strengthens and stretches the lower back and helps to keep the spine in alignment.

Start: Kneel on the floor on all fours. Be sure that your hands are aligned with your shoulders and knees are aligned with your hips. Keep your face down and suck your tummy in.

Movement: Extend your left arm straight out in front of you as you extend your right leg straight out behind you. Lengthen your body from the tip of your left hand fingers to the tip of your right foot toes, as far as possible. (See photo.) Hold for a slow count of 15. Repeat the exercise with right arm and left leg raised.

Tips: Imagine a rope pulling your fingers from the front and another rope pulling your feet from the back. This will aid you in keeping balance. The stretch will feel great. Each breath should be slow and deep.

Options: If you are finding it hard to balance, you can simplify the move by doing the arm and leg movements separately. You can turn this into an advanced move by using a stability ball. Lie on the ball with abs and chest down. Your legs should be straight behind you pressing against the wall to help keep you steady. Stretch your arms out in front of you. Lift your torso a few inches off the ball and hold.

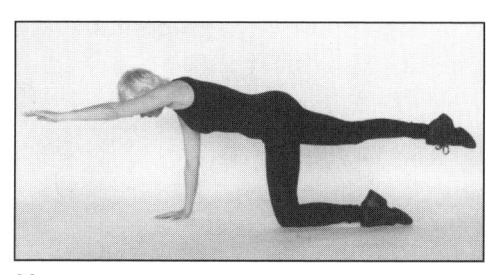

Movement

Stability Ball Extension

This works the lower back and helps to stabilize the middle section of your body.

Start: Lie on the floor with your arms at your sides. Place your heels on top of a stability ball so that your hips and knees are at a 90-degree angle. (See photo.)

Movement: The ball should roll slightly as you extend both legs and hips up. Stay in that position for a slow count to 10. (See photo.) Return to starting position. Work up to 10 repetitions.

Tip: The key is to contract your abdominal muscles and hold your lower back still during the upward position.

Options: Simplify the move by using a chair rather than the stability ball. Increase the difficulty of the move by increasing the length of the hold and/or the repetitions.

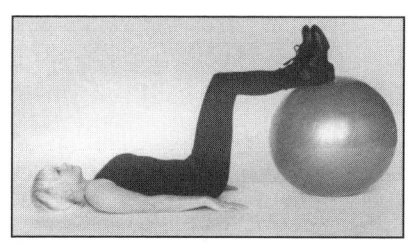

Start

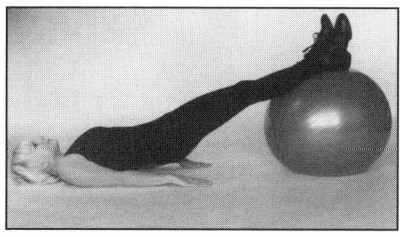

Movement

Hang Straight

This exercise incorporates the lower-back and abdominal muscles.

     Start: On the floor facing downward, balance your weight on your forearms and toes. Elbows should be bent and hands together. Do not raise or drop your head. Keep it in neutral alignment with the rest of your spine.

Movement: Contract your abdominals and keep your back straight. Hold for a slow count of 10. (See photo.) Rest and repeat 5 times.

Tip: Make sure you keep your back flat and do not drop your abs or back. Do not let your butt stick up beyond its natural curve.

Options: If this exercise is too difficult, do the same move but bend your knees and balance on them rather than on your toes. For more of a challenge, increase the length of time you hold the position. It's more difficult than it looks.

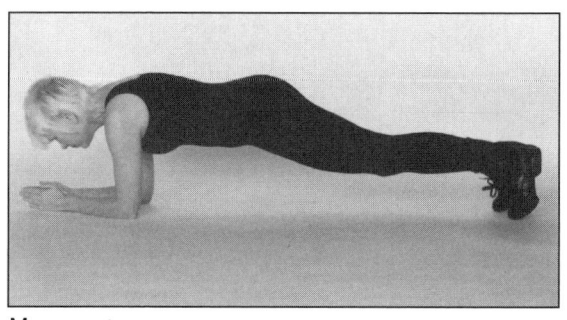

Movement

chapter

5

Cool-Down

After doing such a great job with the *Erase Your Waist* workout, you may feel like collapsing and just leaving out the cool-down. I can totally understand your sentiment, but I strongly advise you not to crash. The next few minutes that you spend cooling down could be the most critical part of your entire workout if you want to achieve fast, maximum results.

When you are doing the *Erase Your Waist* workout, there are a number of physiological changes that occur within your body. For one thing, your body temperature rises and your heart rate goes up. If you don't do the cool-down to recover from the stress on your system, your condition will not progress as well it should and, in fact, could get worse. That's why in some cases you hear people complain about doing ab work and not seeing a change. By doing the cool-down, your body has a chance to adequately recover. It is actually during the recovery phase that muscle changes take place. That is the underlying philosophy of this type of progressive training. You repeatedly move from the workout phase into the recovery phase. Each recovery session will take you to a new level of muscle definition and strength.

The cool-down can benefit a successful recovery in a number of ways. It helps to remove excess acids from the muscles to help you avoid muscle soreness. It also acts as a catalyst in the repair of "micro" tears in your muscle fibers. (This is a normal and necessary occurrence during a workout.) It is the rebuilding of those tears where the sculpting takes place. The cool-down also lowers the body's temperature and helps the heart rate

return to its pre-workout level. Bottom line—by the next workout session, you'll be on your way to a better shape than the last. That in itself makes the cool-down worth it.

Relax

As you begin to incorporate the cool-down into your workout, you will find that this is definitely the "feel good" part of your routine. Enjoy it! You deserve to chill for a moment. As women, we tend to put everyone else first. Use this time to rid yourself of any tension that has built up within you. This time is just for you.

Exercises and Equipment

Following are the cool-down exercises. Enjoy!

1. Standing Lower Back Stretch
2. Knee to Chest
3. Fetal Position Stretch
4. Torso Stretch
5. Back Extensions
6. Cobra
7. Child Pose
8. Prone Position
9. Stand, Breathe, and Reach

Equipment needed:
• Fitness Mat, Towel, or Rug

Standing Lower Back Stretch

This is a great stretch for the lower back. It's a particularly good one if you sit at a desk all day.

Start: Stand with your feet hip-width apart and knees slightly bent. Place your palms on your lower back with your fingers pointing down. Your hands should be resting just above your hips.

Movement: Press your palms into your lower back so that the muscles are stretched. (See photo.) Hold for 30 seconds.

Tip: Remember to keep breathing throughout the stretch.

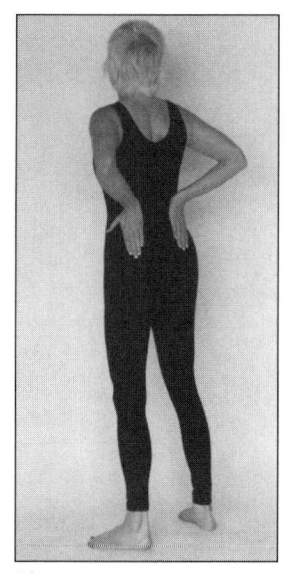

Movement

Knee to Chest

This cool-down exercise stretches the lower back, hamstrings, and hips.

>Start: Lie on the floor on your back with both legs straight out in front of you. Do not tense up.
>
>Movement: Lift your left leg up with your knee bent and pull it to your chest. (See photo.) Hold for 30 seconds. Repeat on the right side.

Tip: Breath deeply throughout the exercise.

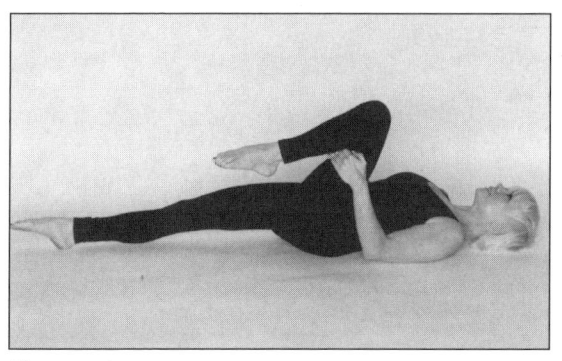

Movement

Fetal Position Stretch

Feel like a baby again with this fetal position lower-back stretch.

Start: Lie on the floor on your back with your knees pressed into your chest.

Movement: Pull your knees as close and tight to your body as possible. (See photo.) Hold up for 30 seconds. Repeat.

Tips: Be sure to keep your upper back on the floor so that you feel the stretch in your lower back. Try doing this move first thing in the morning. It's especially effective if you sleep on your stomach.

Option: This move can also be done in a chair. Simply lift your knees up to your chest and tuck your forehead toward your knees. Try it at the office in between computer tasks.

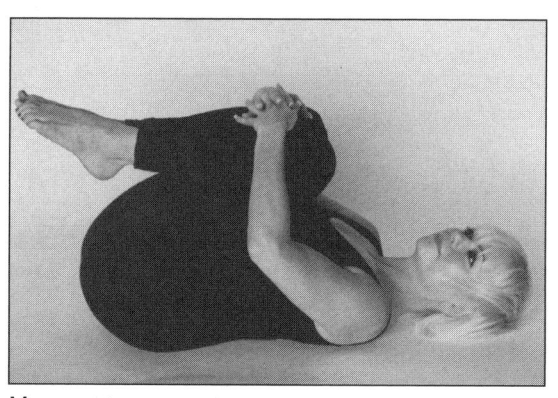

Movement

Torso Stretch

This stretch works the entire spine. It also brings the shoulders and arms into play.

Start: Sit erect on the floor with one leg crossed over the other. Place your hands gently on your knees.

Movement: Bend forward slightly as you bring your left arm up and over to your right side. (See photo.) Hold for 30 seconds. Repeat on the other side.

Tip: Hold your abdominals in to support the lower back.

Options: You can simplify the move by bending forward with no arm lifts. To create more of a challenge, lift both arms up and to the side together.

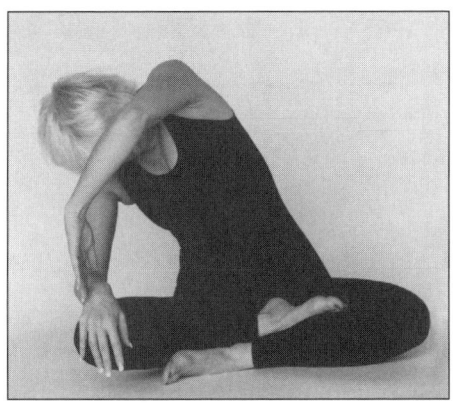

Movement

Back Extensions

This strengthens the lower back and is a perfect compliment to your ab exercises.

Start: Lie face down on the floor with your arms straight out in front of you, palms down, and your legs straight out behind you. Hold your tummy in.

Movement: Lift your left arm and right leg simultaneously just slightly off the floor. Hold for a slow count of 5. (See photo.) Repeat with your right arm and left leg. Do 3 sets of 5 counts on each side.

Tips: Do not do this exercise if you experience pain in your lower back. Exhale during the "lifting" part of the move. Never lift higher than a few inches off the floor.

Options: To make the move more challenging, you can work one side at a time. First lift your left arm and left leg and then lift your right arm and right leg. It is easier to do if you lift only one appendage at a time. First the left arm, and then the right leg, and then the right arm, and then the left leg.

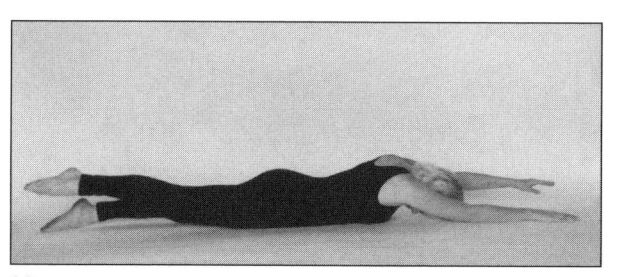

Movement

Cobra

This yoga-inspired move is a favorite of mine. It stretches the abs and elongates the entire spine. In addition to that, it stretches the chest and strengthens the buns and thighs.

Start: Lie on your stomach with your forehead on the floor and your legs straight out behind you. Keep your legs close together. With fingers pointing forward, place your palms to the side and slightly in front of your shoulders. Elbows should be bent and pointing up. Pushing your hands down, lift your chest a tiny bit off the floor.

Movement: Push your palms even harder into the floor as you straighten your arms and lift your upper body as far as you can without feeling pain. Hold for 5 seconds. (See photo.) Repeat.

Tip: To maintain good form, press your hipbones into the floor throughout the entire exercise.

Option: If it's too difficult to press off your palms (e.g. wrist problems) you can press off the forearms. Lift your entire upper body off the floor. Include your arms in the move. Be careful to keep the lower body stable so as not to hurt your back. Make sure those hip bones are still pressed into the floor.

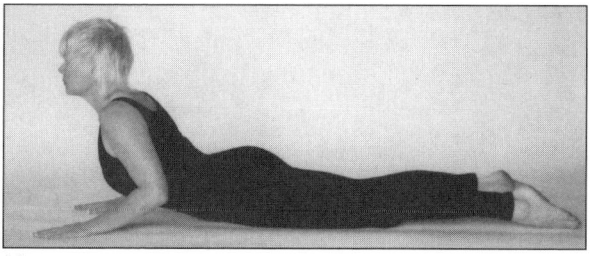

Movement

Child Pose

This is another yoga move that I love—it helps me connect with my inner child. The child pose stretches the entire spine as it relieves tension. Clear your mind of any negative thoughts.

Start: Kneel on the floor with your buns resting on your heels.

Movement: Bend forward from your hips and let your forehead touch the floor. Lengthen your spine but do not tense it up. Let your chest rest on your thighs. Arms should lie limply along your sides. (See photo.) Inhale and exhale very slowly. Feel your rib cage expanding and contracting.

Tip: Focus on your breathing; it should be very slow. Feel your breath through the movement of your rib cage.

Options: If you lack flexibility, try placing a pillow under your ankles to assist you with the move. As you progress, do the move with your arms stretched out in front and your palms up.

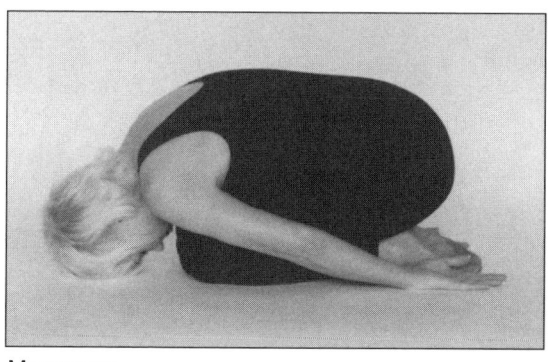

Movement

Prone Position

This is a great wrap-up to a wonderful workout. It helps to calm your mind and relax your body.

Start: Lie on the floor on your stomach so that your face rests on your folded arms. Your legs should be stretched out with toes slightly pointed.

Movement: Breathe slowly and deeply for a minimum of 30 seconds. (See photo.) Close your eyes for total escape.

Tip: Put yourself in the moment. Not a second before or a second after, but in the present time.

Option: If you feel any discomfort, try placing a towel under the trouble spot (e.g., hips).

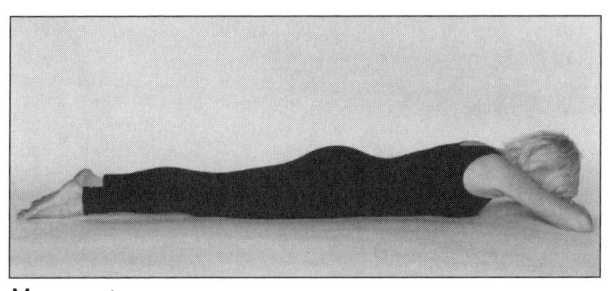

Movement

Stand, Breathe, and Reach

This is the last exercise in the cool-down. It will leave you energized. Stretch with a sense of accomplishment. You did it!

Start: Stand with your feet hip-width apart, knees slightly bent, and arms down at your sides. (See Photo.)

Movement: In one continuous and fluid motion, inhale as you raise your arms up from the sides. (See photo.) Exhale as you bring them back down. Repeat three times.

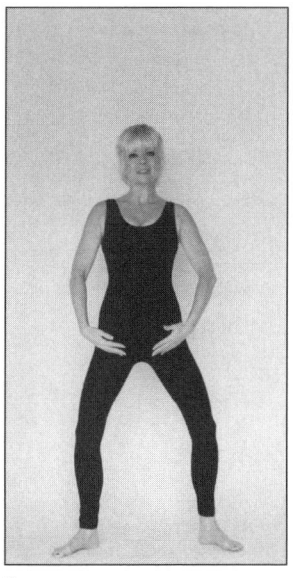

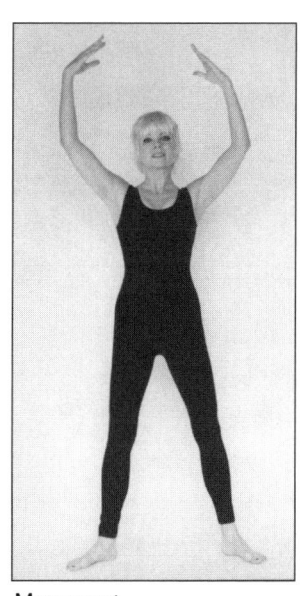

Start

Movement

chapter

6

Posture and Breathing

I confess to being a bit of a stickler when it comes to posture and breathing exercises. I include them in all of my fitness programs, and the *Erase Your Waist* program is no exception. The reason is simple—incorporating good posture and breathing into your routine will produce the quickest results. In fact, if you don't have good posture and proper breathing techniques, you will never achieve the trim, taut tummy you crave. For that reason, I ask you to pay close attention to the posture and breathing skills on which you are about to embark.

Poor Posture Slump

Good posture makes a significant difference in our overall appearance, especially in the torso area. Unfortunately, the lifestyle of many women puts them in the position that I call "poor posture slump." All of us are prone to this preposterous slouch. We spend so much of our lives in a seated position; everything from sitting at a desk or computer to watching television to driving makes the muscles get lazy and cave in. You know the look I'm talking about—droopy shoulders, a bent-over spine, and excess fat hanging out loose over your belt. We might as well add a dozen glazed donuts to the scenario.

I'm sure that vision inspired you to suck it all in and straighten up. Ah ha! We are on to something positive. Start being more aware of your posture. Good posture is not just

the alignment of body parts when you are standing tall in an effort to impress the opposite sex. Posture is how all of your body parts work together whether you are standing, sitting, bending, exercising, or whatever you are doing. It is the way you carry yourself, alone and/or in the company of others.

Your carriage can make or break you. It can affect your whole disposition and the way people respond to you. For example, you can choose to glide into a room like a graceful gazelle, stride in with a strong purpose, or enter with your head and shoulders down, disappearing into oblivion and lonely self-pity. Why not choose a healthy, confident stance? It may not solve all your problems, but at least you will look and feel better.

Posture Check

To achieve good posture, stand with your feet planted on the floor parallel to each other. Your chest should be out and your shoulders back. Not too far back, just enough to slightly lift your breasts up. Be careful not to bring the shoulders up to the ears, which can cause tension. Keep them relaxed. Hold your abdominals in tight and your buttocks tucked under. Pretend you are a marionette being held up from above and below by a tight rope. Don't let that rope go loose, or else your carriage could collapse. Follow these posture perfect tips.

Tips

- Make friends with a full-length mirror. Check yourself from head to toe before you walk out the door. Learn to love your image. Remind yourself to walk tall.
- Elongate the neck and entire spine.
- Keep your chin parallel to the floor. This will help to remove the appearance of a double chin.
- Balance your weight equally on both feet. It helps to point your toes forward. If you point one foot out you may lean too much in one direction, unevenly distributing your weight and throwing you out of alignment.

- Use office and storefront windows as posture check points. It is not vain to glance at your stance in the reflective glass. It's part of healthy posture awareness.
- Do not beat yourself up if you keep catching yourself in the "poor posture slump." Be patient. Old habits take time to change, but with practice you can do it.

Instant Non-Surgical Tummy Tuck

The beauty of good posture is that it can act as an instant non-surgical tummy tuck. That's right! Holding yourself erect can give you the appearance of being ten pounds slimmer in that hard-to-reach middle area. Use good posture to slice inches off your waist without surgery. Try it right now in front of a mirror. See what I mean? You look ten pounds skinnier. What do you think they do in all those before and after advertisements? Couple the instant success of good posture with the *Erase Your Waist* program and you are on your way to a beautiful, taut tummy.

Diaphragmatic Breathing

When it comes to doing an abdominal workout, proper breathing is especially important. Certainly, it can expedite the rate at which you get results. However, there is much more to this breathing story. Holding your breath and/or improper breathing during an abdominal workout can actually build bigger stomach muscles. Yikes! This could be why you or other women you know have gotten frustrated with ab work and have given up in the past. Not to worry. Let me share my tips on proper breathing. They are an integral part of the *Erase Your Waist* program.

Holding your stomach in provides an excellent natural girdle and can make you appear slimmer. The problem occurs when you keep your stomach so tightly pulled in, without allowing for a natural breath movement, that the breath is erroneously shifted into the thoracic (upper chest) cavity. In time, improper breathing patterns are developed. This can

affect your health and appearance, and your tummy exercises will not be as effective. Let's check out what type of breathing pattern you should be using.

Start by resting your hands underneath your rib cage, with your fingers close together and pointing in toward your belly button. When you inhale, your stomach should force your hands out sideways and your fingers will automatically open up as the diaphragm (thin muscular membrane that divides the chest and belly) drops. As you exhale, your hands should return back in. This is what is called diaphragmatic breathing. Use it in exercise. Use it in life.

Tip: Be sure to breathe using the diaphragm. Many women make the mistake of primarily using their chests to breathe, which is called thoracic breathing.

Breathing Check Exercises

Below are the breathing check exercises. They provide a great foundation for the *Erase Your Waist* program and will, in fact, enhance all your fitness work. Don't minimize their importance.

1. Lying Down Breath Check
2. Standing Up Breath Check

Lying Down Breath Check

This will help you establish excellent breathing patterns. You will need four medium size books.

      Start: Lie flat on your back on the floor with arms outstretched to the sides. Place four books directly over your abdomen. (See photo.)
Movement: Inhale slowly as you let the books rise up. Pause at the top. (See photo.) Exhale as you slowly lower the books back to start. Repeat 3 times.

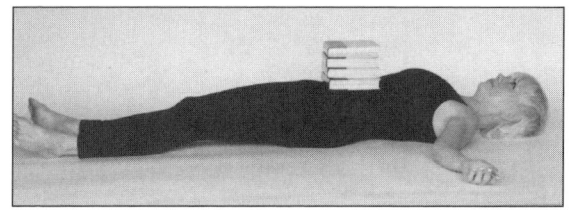

Start

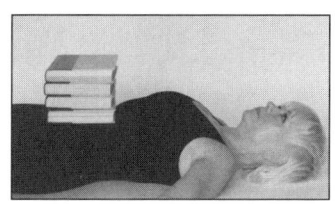

Movement

Standing Up Breath Check

This exercise will help you develop the skill of diaphragmatic breathing. I recommend that you use it throughout the day. It will help you incorporate it into your very being.

> Start: Stand with your feet hip-width apart. Place your hands under your rib cage. (See photo.)
>
> Movement: Slowly inhale as you use the breath in your abdomen to push your hands out to the side. (See photo.) Slowly exhale as your hands return to starting position. Repeat 3 times.

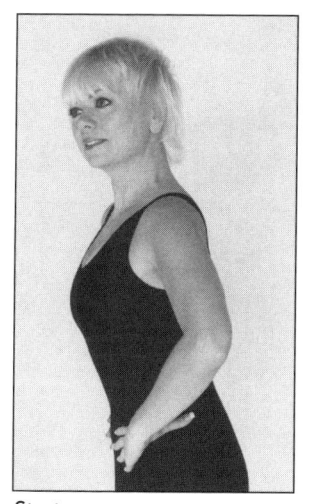

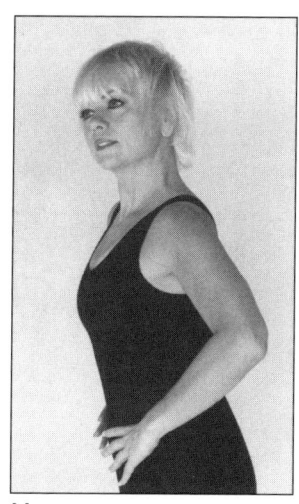

Start

Movement

Posture Check Exercises

Try these posture check exercises. They will enhance your stance and improve the look of your midsection.

1. The Beauty Pageant Posture Walk
2. Chair Hold
3. Shoulder Blade Squeeze
4. Vertebrae Alignment

The Beauty Pageant Posture Walk

When I was a little girl, I loved to pretend I was Miss America. I'd put a crown on my head and wave to my adoring fans. Part of the fantasy included the beauty pageant posture walk. You may giggle about personal memories of yourself or a friend strutting down an imaginary runway, but one can't deny the real-life posture benefits that come from a tall and regal walk. Take a moment of escape to be queen of your own private kingdom in this fun exercise.

Start: Balance a book on top of your head.

Movement: Stand tall and erect as you gracefully walk around the room trying not to drop the book off your head. (See photos.) This old-fashioned move gets a big thumbs-up. (Waving to your imaginary audience is optional.)

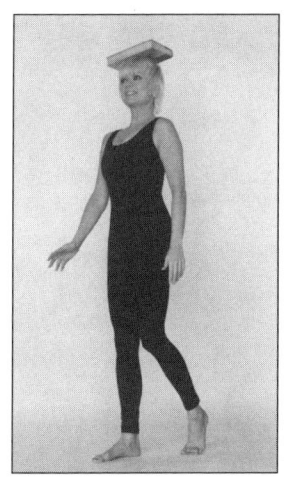

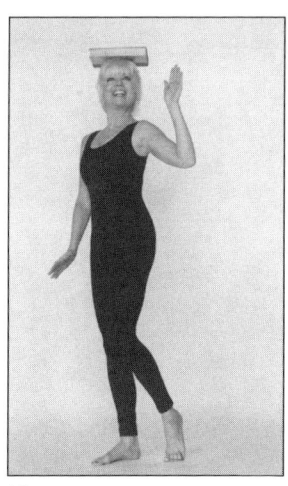

Movement

Movement

Chair Hold

This is a great posture exercise that is superb for the back. It also works the front of your thighs and quadriceps.

     Start: Stand with your back against the wall. Push the small of your back into the wall as you lower yourself into a chair position. (See photo.)
Movement: Hold for 10 seconds; eventually work up to 30 seconds, and then a minute or more.

Tips: Do not arch your back. Keep your legs in a 90-degree angle.

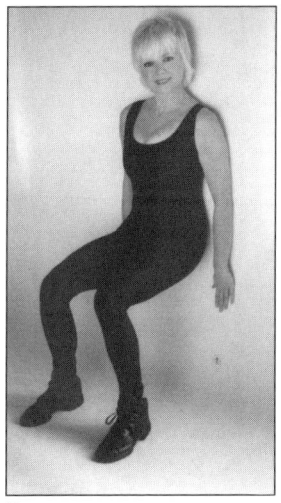

Start

Shoulder Blade Squeeze

Great posture exercise with emphasis on the mid-back.

Start: Sit or stand tall. Interlace your fingers behind your head with elbows outstretched to the sides.

Movement: Squeeze the shoulder blades together. (See photo.) Hold for a count of 5. Relax. Repeat 3 times.

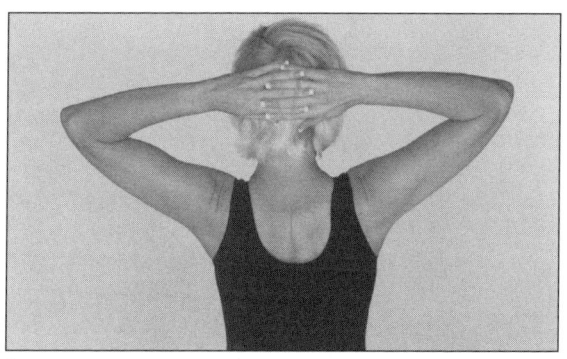

Start

Vertebrae Alignment

This is a subtle but very effective posture move, employed by many physical therapists.

- **Start:** Stand in an upright position. Maintain good posture. Place two fingers above your upper lip. (See photo.)
- **Movement:** Gently push your head straight back without raising your head up or down. Keep the chin parallel to the floor. (See photo.) Hold for a count of 5. Return to start. Relax. Repeat 3 times.

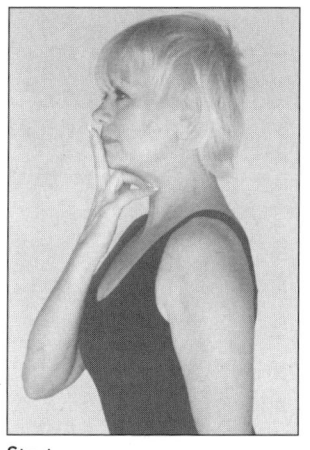

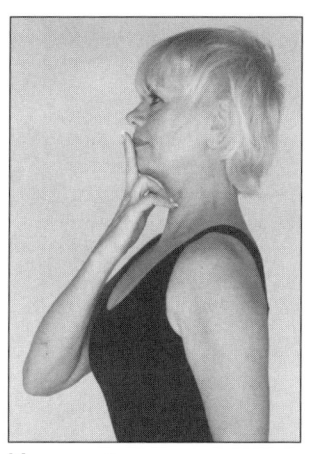

Start

Movement

chapter

7

Nutrient Knowledge

It's funny how some people love to watch what I eat. It's as if they expect me to live on soybeans, celery, and carrot sticks alone. I certainly enjoy these foods, but heaven forbid I should get caught eating a scrumptious shortbread cookie or a decadent piece of creamy milk chocolate. Truth be told, I love to eat and refuse to deny myself the palatable pleasures of a wide range of epicurean delights. Does that mean I'm one of those chicks who can scarf up everything in sight without gaining an ounce? Not!

I maintain a healthy weight because I exercise regularly and am able to make good, healthy, educated food choices. Sure, I indulge sometimes, but I make an informed decision about every morsel of food that enters my mouth. In this chapter, I will give you scientific information on no-nonsense nutrients. You will have the tools necessary to take charge of your own dietary choices. Digest these food facts and you can escape the consequences of being nutritionally challenged.

Knowing about nutrients will help take some of the confusion out of food choices. All food is made up of a mixture of six major nutrients. Your body is also made up of those same six nutrients. That explains why the saying, "You are what you eat!" is so meaningful.

There are three nutrients that are essential to our body but provide no energy or calories: vitamins, minerals, and water.

There are three other nutrients that do have energy or calories: fat, protein, and carbohydrates. One gram of protein is equal to four calories, one gram of carbohydrate is equal to four calories, and one gram of fat is equal to nine calories. Don't spend your energy (calories) dwelling on which of these nutrients is "good" for you and which is "bad" for you. All six of them play an integral part in the way our systems function.

Water

Water is a wonderful nutrient. Besides oxygen, it is our most important life-sustaining element. It makes up about 50 to 70 percent of our body's weight. Contrary to what most people think, the bodies of lean people have a relatively higher percentage of water than people with high body fat. Water comprises 75 percent of our muscle tissue and 25 percent of our fat tissue. Perhaps that's why in Hollywood, where thin is in, water has become the drink of choice. (You should see my car; I'm embarrassed to admit how many water bottles are piled up in the passenger seat.)

The traditional advice to drink eight glasses of water a day is still very sound. Unfortunately, when people get thirsty, they often opt for other beverages. Most Americans don't even come close to drinking a healthy amount of water.

There are many excellent reasons to drink plenty of water. It regulates your body temperature and aids in digestion. It helps to keep your skin clear and healthy. It protects the cells in your body, and can rid you of constipation and even irritability. The big bonus is that it can help with weight loss—water naturally curbs your appetite. Plus, the very act of drinking water burns more calories through digestion than you consume, since there are no calories in water! Consider it a mini workout that you can do while sitting on your couch.

Urologists will tell you that water helps to dissolve calcium in the urine, which can help to prevent kidney stones. It also helps to ward off urinary infection. They recommend checking your urine color to test if you are drinking enough water. If

your urine is dark colored, then you need to increase your intake of H_2O.

All women should drink water, but for some it is especially critical. If you are pregnant, a nursing mother, or very active in sports, you need to drink up. Studies show that women in careers where they serve others—such as teachers, nurses, or flight attendants—are more likely to forget to sip water. It's a good idea to have a cup of water with every meal and add in several cups between meals.

With regards to exercise, I'm going to recommend that you drink water before, during, and after. Drink eight ounces of water a half-hour before exercise, three ounces of water every ten minutes during exercise, and another eight ounces after exercise. Do not let thirst be an indicator of when to drink fluids. By the time you feel the need to drink water, your body could already be entering a state of dehydration. Drinking water during exercise will significantly reduce the stress on your system and improve your fitness.

Vitamins

Vitamins are organic nutrients essential to life. They play a starring role in the production of energy, in growth, and in regulating your body's metabolism. They help to speed up chemical reactions in the body—and the list goes on. Since the body does not manufacture them, they must be obtained from food. Vitamins have no calories.

There are thirteen vitamins. They can be separated into two different types: the fat-soluble and the water-soluble.

Fat-Soluble Vitamins

Vitamins A, D, E, and K are fat-soluble, which means that excess amounts are stored in fat. Heads-up, dear reader: As necessary and beneficial as these vitamins are, they require a word of caution. Taken in excessive amounts, they can be toxic. That's why if you take over-the-counter supplements, be sure to read the labels so that you don't self-medicate

inappropriately. Instead, I encourage you to fill up on fabulous foods that are naturally loaded with these vitamins.

Following is a list of fat-soluble vitamins, what they do, the adult U.S. Recommended Daily Allowance (RDA) measured in International Units (IU), and sources for each.

Vitamin A
- Helps the growth of skin, bones, and teeth. Plays a key role in vision.
- U.S. RDA is 5,000 IU.
- Found in deep green leafy vegetables (e.g., spinach), yellow-orange fruits and vegetables (e.g., carrots, sweet potatoes, apricots, cantaloupe).

Vitamin D
- Aids in bone and tooth formation. Helps the body utilize calcium and phosphorous. Helps maintain the heart and nervous system.
- U.S. RDA is 400 IU.
- Found in fortified milk, eggs, dairy products, fish; the body can also synthesize vitamin D when the skin is exposed to sunlight.

Vitamin E
- Supports blood cells and essential fatty acids.
- U.S. RDA is 30 IU.
- Found in multigrain cereals, nuts, seeds, green leafy vegetables.

Vitamin K
- Aids in blood clotting action.
- U.S. RDA has not been established yet.
- Found in grains, green leafy vegetables, cabbage, cauliflower, soybeans.

Water-Soluble Vitamins

Water-soluble vitamins, unlike fat-soluble ones, are absorbed in the body's water. That means that if you have an excess amount in your system, they can be excreted. Water-soluble vitamins consist of vitamin C and the B vitamins.

Following is a list of key water-soluble vitamins, what they do, the adult U.S. Recommended Daily Allowance (RDA) in milligrams, and sources for each.

Vitamin C
- Essential for bones, blood vessels, muscles. Aids in iron absorption.
- U.S. RDA is 60 mg.
- Found in citrus fruits, cantaloupe, vegetables (e.g., tomatoes, broccoli, greens, sweet potatoes).

B1 (Thiamine)
- Important for your body metabolism, growth, and muscle tone.
- U.S. RDA is 1.5 mg.
- Found in oatmeal, whole grains, rice, liver, dried beans, soybeans.

B2 (Riboflavin)
- Important for good skin, prevents light sensitivity in the eyes, helps with metabolizing of carbohydrates.
- U.S. RDA is 1.7 mg.
- Found in whole grains, organ meats, green leafy vegetables.

B3 (Niacin)
- Plays a role in the metabolizing of protein, carbohydrates, and fat.
- U.S. RDA is 20 mg.
- Found in nuts, lean meats, poultry, fish, dairy products, eggs, wheat bread.

B6 (Pyridoxine)
- Metabolizes protein and contributes to healthy tissues.
- U.S. RDA is 2 mg.
- Found in bananas, prunes, fish, poultry.

B12 (Cobalamin)
- Helps the neurological system, also works in the metabolizing of fat and protein.
- U.S. RDA 6 micrograms.
- Found in fish, dairy products, meats.

Biotin
- Helps to metabolize protein, fat, and carbohydrates.
- U.S. RDA is .3 mg.
- Found in legumes, whole grains, eggs, fish, dairy products, broccoli, cabbage, potatoes.

Folate
- Contributes to our genetic makeup. Helps to produce red blood cells.
- U.S. RDA is .4 mg.
- Found in lentils, green leafy vegetables.

Pantothenic Acid
- Aids in enzyme reactions in the body.
- U.S. RDA is 10 mg.
- Found in legumes, whole grains, lean meats, fruits, and vegetables.

Vitamin Summary

If you want a tight tummy and good health, you need to incorporate vitamins in the *Erase Your Waist* program. I just gave you a lot of details, but basically, it's important to eat a varied diet with plenty of whole grains, fresh fruits and vegetables, and low-fat dairy products. Remember that excess fat-soluble vitamins are retained in fat and excess water-soluble vitamins are

excreted. Revisit the list of vitamins I gave you from time to time. Make a conscientious effort to put variety in your meal planning. Include a supplement if necessary. You will find that vitamin intake will become a natural part of your healthy life-style.

Minerals

Minerals are another requirement of good nutrition. They do everything from regulating your heartbeat to transferring oxygen to every cell. They play a role in the development of bones and teeth, and regulate water retention. Minerals support practically all of our body's functions.

There are two types of minerals: major and minor. Major minerals are defined as those that you need to consume in amounts over 100 milligrams a day. They include calcium, phosphorous, sodium, chloride, magnesium, and potassium. Our bodies need only "trace" amounts of the minor minerals, which include zinc, iron, copper, iodine, manganese, molybdenum, arsenic, boron, nickel, vanadium, chromium, selenium, fluoride, and silicon. Don't be fooled. Just because we only need trace amounts does not make these any less important than the major minerals. We need both types.

Whole books are written on individual minerals. There's so much conflicting information it's enough to put you in a state of mineral madness. Take a breath! To simplify things for the *Erase Your Waist* program, I'm going to make a few recommendations. As I've stated earlier, include a lot of variety in your diet. I'll explain how to do that in more detail in chapter 8. As a woman, you should also monitor your calcium intake carefully. The U.S. RDA is 1,000 milligrams a day.

A Word on Supplements

The jury is still out on whether supplements help or not. There are just as many experts who recommend them as there are who condemn them. More research certainly needs to be done. One thing that the vast majority agree on is that supplements are not a supplement for a balanced diet. This puts you in the

driver's seat once again. Take charge. If you feel you are not getting the recommended levels of vitamins and minerals in your meals, supplements could be helpful. Just be sure that you read the labels to be sure that you are not getting toxic amounts of any one vitamin. I would also advise you always to let your physician know of any supplements that you are taking.

Protein

These days, proteins have been the focus of a great deal of media attention. The truth is that proteins have always been an integral part of a balanced diet. After all, they are the building blocks of cells and tissues in our body. We need them for many body functions including immune system functioning, fluid balance, blood clotting, and hormone production, to name a few.

If you were to look at proteins in a lab, you would see that they are made up of a chain of amino acids. Picture oxygen, hydrogen, carbon, and nitrogen hooked up together. It's the nitrogen in that connection that makes proteins different from carbohydrates or fats. That's why a protein molecule is so much bigger than a carbohydrate or fat molecule. Cool, huh?

The amino acids are divided into two types: essential and nonessential. There are twenty amino acids that we need in order to live. Eleven are termed nonessential because the body can manufacture them on its own. The other nine are termed essential and must be consumed through your diet.

Here's the scoop. You can get all nine essential amino acids in animal foods. They are called complete proteins. If you are the carnivorous kind—go for it! This, however, does not give you carte blanche to order a side of beef at every meal—portion-size does come into play.

Vegetarian foods lack one or more essential proteins and so they are considered incomplete proteins. If you are a vegetarian, you will need to be a little more careful when trying to consume your essential amino acids. I advise you to learn about combining foods to make up complete proteins (consult a good

vegetarian cookbook that addresses the subject). For example, beans and rice work great together because grains and legumes can make up complete proteins. They are beneficial even if not eaten together, as long as you consume them on the same day.

Whether you eat meat or are a vegetarian, protein needs to be part of your diet. After water, it is the most abundant substance in your body. That does not mean you should go into protein overload—in fact, too much protein can be damaging. The exact amount of protein necessary in a healthy diet is an issue that continues to be debated among experts. You are safe if you keep your protein intake to about 10-15 percent of your daily calories.

Carbohydrates

Carbohydrates are another popular buzzword on the nutrition circuit. Somehow, they are always categorized either "good" or "bad." Do we have to be on either bandwagon? Carbs are a major source of energy. They charge up every cell in your system like the Energizer Bunny. Technically, they are a combination of oxygen, hydrogen, and carbon atoms. These atoms bond together to form sugars, starches, or fiber. Any way you look at it, carbohydrates should be a staple of your diet.

The carbohydrate confusion sometimes takes place because many people do not differentiate between the two types of carbohydrates. There are complex carbohydrates (whole-grain breads and cereals, rice, pasta) and simple sugars (soda, cake, cookies). Once inside your body, all carbohydrates are turned into glucose. Glucose is what the cells use to provide your body with all the energy it needs to perform its countless functions.

Does that mean you should fill up on candy bars under the guise of getting an energy fix? Sorry—no. Candy bars are made up of simple sugars that quickly enter the blood stream. If they raise your blood sugar level too high, you will be left with an excess amount of glucose. You might as well

paste that candy bar on your tummy, because the excess glucose will change into fat and be stored in a fat cell. As a woman, you have normal fat cells throughout your body, including a concentration of them on your stomach, which the excess glucose will plump right up if you eat too many simple sugars. That only makes it harder to trim the abdominal area.

Complex carbohydrates are different from simple sugars. They are better for you because it takes them longer to break down in your system. The calories you consume from complex carbohydrates are more likely to be used up as energy rather than stored on your stomach or elsewhere as fat. The other benefit of complex carbohydrates is that they are packed with nutrients. A candy bar doesn't offer you much other than sugar. In general, your diet should consist of 55–60 percent carbohydrates, the majority of which should be complex carbohydrates.

Fat

Don't feel bad. You, I, and most other women don't like to think about fat—or more accurately, we think about it too much. In a perfect world, I would like to eat as many fatty foods as I want without gaining an ounce or hurting my health. Unfortunately, that fantasy will never happen. Fat is not all bad, though. We certainly need it for survival. Perhaps it is my love/hate relationship with fat that has given me the incentive to win the waist-weight-gain war. Let me help you understand fat so that you can start being more selective about meal planning. There are fabulous foods you can choose to fill you up. This information can make a significant difference in the results of the *Erase Your Waist* program.

Fat, like carbohydrates, supplies your body with energy to perform its many activities. It ensures proper growth in children and transports fat-soluble vitamins throughout the body. It also enhances food texture and is partly responsible for the flavor and the aroma of food. No wonder we are all so fond of fat.

You have probably heard the terms "good" fats and "bad" fats, which have become popular with dietitians and food corporations. I use the terms as well. They have helped me develop a healthy attitude about eating. Although I do splurge on bad fats occasionally, the majority of my fat calories come from good fats.

Monounsaturated and polyunsaturated fats are considered the good fats. Foods that contain these types of fat include olives, olive and canola oil, avocados, salmon, tuna, walnuts, and peanut oil. Saturated fats and trans fats are considered the bad fats. Foods that contain these types of fat include ice cream, beef, butter, margarine, processed foods, and mayonnaise.

Much has been in the news lately about the bad trans fats. These are polyunsaturated oils that are saturated with hydrogen atoms. Food corporations love trans fats because they help foods have a longer shelf life. They are usually labeled as hydrogenated or partially hydrogenated, which could fool the unsuspecting consumer into eating bad fat. In the near future, companies may be required to label trans fats as such, making them easier to identify.

Research shows that too much fat can lead to heart disease and put you at risk for some cancers. It does not help your cholesterol level, either. Let's not forget that it can also ruin all the wonderful work you are doing in the *Erase Your Waist* routine. It is generally recommended that about 20 to 25 percent of your caloric intake come from fat (remember, a gram of fat has more calories than a gram of protein or carbohydrate). The American Heart Association advises no more than 30 percent.

Since I enjoy food, I have a personal tip that helps me not to go overboard on fat. I make a conscientious effort to include good fats in my meal planning. I find that they fill me up and I don't feel deprived. Many people who avoid fat altogether are starving themselves and end up pigging out on the bad fats. Did you ever eat a pint of ice cream in one sitting? I rest my case.

chapter 8

Nutritionally Yours

This chapter will provide you with excellent array of realistic weight management tips and nutrition information. Whether to diet or not, pyramid power, food journals, label reading, serving sizes, etc., are important topics to understand when you're are striving to Erase Your Waist. It's up to you to exercise your power of choice as to what you want to credit to your personal health account. I have delivered the message—now it's nutritionally yours. Embrace this knowledge and take charge!

To Diet or Not

Every time I turn around, there's a new diet on the market. High protein, high carbohydrate, high fat, cabbage, grapefruit—the list goes on and on. It can be overwhelming. If you think I'm going to recommend some fad diet in this book, you can forget about it. Diets don't work. Sensible food consumption is the answer.

What determines sensible eating? I personally preach a very individualized plan based on your specific needs as a woman. We are all different. What works for one woman may not work for another. When you take into account medical variances such as diabetes, hypoglycemia, or any number of health-related factors, cookie-cutter diets don't cut it. That's why I think it's irresponsible for an author to make a blanket statement in a book about a diet plan that is supposed to work for everybody.

Rather, I challenge you to take charge of your own body. Read all the information you can about healthy living. Talk with your registered dietitian and health care provider about your personal needs. Only then will you be able to make an informed decision about your food choices.

That being said, there are basic nutritional needs common to everybody, and clinically proven information that will help you achieve a healthier lifestyle. You're not alone if you feel clueless on this subject. Most people know a few nutritional buzzwords, but that's it. Fortunately, it's never too late to keep learning. You will discover that there is a cornucopia of foods that will satiate your appetite without causing inappropriate weight gain. Fear not—hunger or starvation has no place in the *Erase Your Waist* program.

Pyramid Power and Beyond

There is much to be said about the relevance of water, minerals, vitamins, proteins, carbohydrates, and fats. We can't live without them. You need to make sure you are getting the right amount of nutrients. How can you be sure? Well, you can carry a calculator in your purse and measure grams, micrograms, calories, etc. There's nothing wrong with that, except it's not very practical or much fun for those of us who aren't into numbers. Fortunately, the USDA introduced the pyramid we all know today. There are some experts who would like to rearrange it. In fact, there's much talk about making it more specific. As this is being printed, new guidelines are being established. For example, why not show a better representation of fats that are actually good for you? I look forward enthusiastically to these changes. For now, however, the pyramid offers you a basic breakdown of the food groups with guidelines to help you make personal healthy dietary choices.

Many women have seen the pyramid and know it's supposed to be good for them but don't really understand it at all. Let me assure you that if you don't totally get it, you are not alone. Once and for all, let's clarify the power of the pyramid.

The food guide pyramid was published in 1992 after much research. It separates food into five major groups, plus an additional segment for fats, oils, and sweets. If you take the time to understand the food groups a little better, you will be able to trim your waist and if you choose, you can eliminate that bulky calculator from your purse.

Bread, Cereal, Rice, and Pasta
This is the largest food group at the bottom of the pyramid. The USDA recommends six to eleven servings a day. Some people try to give this group a bad rap. Upon close inspection of this segment, you will find that it has many nutrient-rich foods. You will also find it includes foods that are high in fat. It's a matter of making an educated choice. Let's take a look at some healthy but tasty options.

Grains

Erase Your Waist Choice	Try To Avoid
Whole grains	Buttery snack crackers
Hot cereal	Croissants
Plain noodle pastas	Doughnuts
Dried peas and beans	Pasta with cream sauce

Fruit Group
Above the bread, cereal, rice, and pasta group is the fruit group. It certainly is one of my favorites. The USDA recommends two to four servings a day. I find that a piece of fresh fruit often will satisfy a craving for sweets. When I was a little girl, we had a peach tree in our yard. My mom would freeze sliced peaches. Yummy! They were better than any fattening dessert could ever be.

Fruit

Erase Your Waist Choice	Try To Avoid
Medium size apple, orange, or pear	Fruits canned in heavy syrup
4 oz. orange, apple, or grapefruit juice	Fruity drinks
1 cup of blueberries or strawberries	Limit fruit juice to no more than 4 oz. per serving

Vegetable Group

The other group above the bread, cereal, rice, and pasta group is the vegetable group. The USDA recommends three to five servings a day. You won't find any reputable nutrition expert who negates the value of vegetables. There are so many different kinds that are jam-packed with nutrients. It's fun to peruse the grocery store aisles in search of a new vegetable to try.

Vegetables

Erase Your Waist Choice	Try To Avoid
Green leafy vegetables	Butter or cream sauce on vegetables
Carrots	
Broccoli	
Vegetable juice	
Lemon juice or spices instead of sauce	

Meat, Poultry, Fish, Dry Beans, Eggs, and Nuts Groups

The USDA recommends two to three servings a day. It's very easy to fill up on foods from these groups. I say—Enjoy! Just

remember that moderation is a key element in making the *Erase Your Waist* program work. Be careful not to choose foods that are deep fried or high in saturated fats. Contrary to a recent misleading advertisement, fried chicken from fast food restaurants is not a healthy choice, even if it *is* low in carbohydrates.

Meat

Erase Your Waist Choice	Try To Avoid
Lean meats (trim fat)	Fatty cuts of meat
Beef	Duck
Poultry (no skin)	Organ meats
Fish	Sausage
Shellfish	Hot dogs

Milk, Yogurt, and Cheese
The USDA recommends two to three servings a day. I suggest you choose fat-free items from this group. That way you will get good nutrients and avoid all the saturated fat.

Dairy

Erase Your Waist Choice	Try To Avoid
Low-fat and non-fat cheese	A whole ice cream cake in one sitting
Skim or low-fat milk	Whole milk and cream
Low-fat yogurt	
Low-fat cottage cheese	

Fats, Oils, and Sweets

This is the tiny segment that we see at the top of the pyramid. The message is use sparingly. These include the foods that are high in fats and simple sugars, e.g., cakes, pies, cookies, etc. If you are overloading on calories from this category, you probably already know it because you have the extra girth around the middle to prove it. It's okay to have a treat on occasion, but if you are finally serious about choosing to be your personal best, remember the phrase, *use sparingly*.

The USDA does not even recommend a serving amount for this category. I realize that you may feel depressed about having to cut back on sweets or hidden fat from this segment. Let me make a suggestion—make the positive change gradually. For example, fat intake should never be higher than 30 percent of your daily calories. If it is significantly higher and you try to cut back all at once, you are setting yourself up for failure. Why not start out as a winner and cut back a more realistic 5 percent of your fat intake at a time? That is a much safer way to manage your weight. The big secret is that it will help you Erase Your Waist for life and have an all-around healthier core, inside and out.

All Calories Are Not Created Equal

The calorie is a unit of energy. It's one of those words that may have crept into your lexicon of guilt-ridden concepts—yet we thrive on calories. They are the fuel for everything our bodies do. Embrace the need for caloric nourishment, and feel good about the pleasures of food. That, of course, does not negate the fact that many people embrace calories a little too much. You will find that as you take charge of your calorie intake, it will be a little easier if you realize that all calories are not created equal.

As I mentioned in chapter 7, carbohydrates and protein contains four calories per gram, while one gram of fat contains nine calories. You are probably familiar with this fact. What you may not realize is that one calorie of one food type

can be more fattening than one calorie of another food type. Let me explain. When you eat carbohydrates or proteins, 20 percent of those calories are used up as energy in the digestive process. Fat, on the other hand, digests easily and therefore uses up only 3 percent of the calories in the digestive process. How does this relate to you? Simply put, 97 percent of a fat calorie ends up stored in the fat cells on your stomach or elsewhere in your body.

I had a client, let's call her Beth, who came to me one day in a tizzy. She couldn't understand why she was not losing any weight. She was doing what appeared to be all the right stuff. She was getting an adequate amount of exercise and taking in the proper amount of calories for her age, frame, and body type. I had Beth keep track of her food intake with a journal so that we could study her records. Ah ha! There it was in her register. Beth had a penchant for late-night ice cream and often had fatty snacks throughout the day. She didn't have too many calories in her diet, but the ones she had were the wrong kind. She was cutting out more nutritional foods in an effort to satisfy her sweet tooth. Her rationale was that as long as she didn't go over the prescribed calorie count, she could eat anything she wanted. Not only did this affect her weight, but she was lacking in many essential nutrients. I had her revisit the food pyramid to be sure she was getting nourishment from all the food groups. A treat is fine on occasion, but the *Erase Your Waist* program is about a healthy balance. That holds true in the *type* of calories you choose.

Serving Size

Portion control plays a big part in the *Erase Your Waist* program. If the USDA recommends six to eleven servings from the bread, cereal, rice, and pasta group, that does not mean you can have super-size fries with every meal. A serving of meat does not equate with a ten-ounce steak. One serving of meat is three ounces—about the size of a deck of cards. One serving of yogurt is eight ounces. When you review the

pyramid for the amount of servings that are required for each group, do not go overboard on the serving size.

I can personally share an ongoing joke I have with one of my best friends. Knowing that I enjoy a good cup of coffee in the morning, she gave me a mug so big I could fit a whole pot of coffee into it. She tried to convince me that, "It's just one cup." Just like you, sometimes I need to take charge and exercise restraint—in this case, by limiting my caffeine intake. Don't be fooled by serving size slip-ups!

Alcohol Consumption

Some people enjoy alcohol for a number of reasons. It could be social, relaxation, or even to escape reality. I'm not going to tell you never to have a drink. Just remember that alcohol is a drug. If you drink, I suggest you use moderation. For women, that is no more than one drink a day, and for men, no more than two drinks per day.

As you continue to take charge of what you put into your system, be aware that alcohol has no essential nutrients. It contains seven calories per gram. Protein and carbohydrates have four calories per gram. A twelve-ounce can of beer gives you one hundred fifty calories and no nutrients. There are about eighty to one hundred calories in a four ounce glass of wine.

If you drink, you should be aware of the amount of alcohol you consume. Again, you must consider serving size. Here is a helpful tip: don't be fooled by glass sizes. Some short glasses actually hold more alcohol than a tall glass. Research proves that the naked eye is easily fooled when it comes to perceived shapes. For example, triangles are thought to be larger than squares and squares are thought to be larger than circles, when all of them are actually equal in volume. Next time you pour yourself a drink or order one, be sure to think twice about the short and tall of it. This valuable information can be applied to any beverage you select.

Food Journal

Many experts believe that keeping a food journal can help you to manage weight, and I agree. According to nationally-known registered dietitian Sandy Gloss, "Many times if you have a weight problem, you are not paying attention to what you are eating. The journal gives you something tangible to look back on. Self-monitoring is one of the most important keys to successful weight loss and management." Gloss suggests you start by keeping a little notebook handy in your pocket. She said, "I'm always telling people, no sheet no eat....Be sure to include in your journal those little snacks that add up....If you don't have time to write it down, then you must not have time to eat it." Gloss recommends that you write down not only what you eat, but how much.

Gloss also points out that different things trigger people to eat different foods. You can learn a lot by periodically documenting feelings, emotions, and activities related to eating. According to Gloss, "Once you identify the problem, then you can start correcting it." Now is a great time to start!

Food Labels

As every "take charge" girl knows, when you go shopping you have to read those labels. Thanks to the Nutrition Labeling and Education Act of 1990 (NLEA), most foods are required to have a visible nutrient label. Initially, the purpose of the act was to help Americans achieve a more balanced diet. It also encouraged food corporations to produce nutritionally sound products. The hope was that advertisers could not get away with false claims. Take advantage of the NLEA every chance you get. I read labels regularly. If I can save a few calories here and a few fat grams there, I'm a happy camper. You should get used to reading food labels, too.

Certainly, food labeling was a big plus that came out of the '90s. Let's look at an example of how you can use that information when deciding which snack is the right choice for you. Following is the information from two nutrition labels. I

personally went to the grocery store and carefully selected two different but comparable snacks. My selections were cherry ice cream and cherry non-fat yogurt. Take a look at the two different labels displayed in the illustration below.

	Cherry Ice Cream	Cherry Non-fat Yogurt
Serving size	1/2 cup	1/2 cup
Calories	260	70
Total fat	16 g	0 g
Saturated fat	11 g	0 g
Cholesterol	70 mg	0 mg
Carbohydrates	26 g	13 g
Sugars	23 g	9 g
Protein	4 g	4 g

Upon close inspection, it's fascinating to see the significant differences in the number comparisons. The ice cream contains over three times the calories of the non-fat yogurt. Of course the non-fat yogurt has no fat, while the ice cream has sixteen grams of fat, eleven of which are saturated. The non-fat yogurt also has no cholesterol and thirteen grams of carbohydrates, while the ice cream has seventy milligrams of cholesterol and twenty-five grams of carbohydrates. They both have four grams of protein.

Common sense would lead one to believe that non-fat yogurt is the better choice. It certainly has more nutritional value. Does that mean you are a bad person if you have ice cream once in a while? I think not. Moderation is the salvation for many of us who love food but want to live healthy.

Just remember to read those labels carefully. In our example, one serving is half a cup—not the whole pint. Even if you choose the non-fat yogurt because of its nutritional value, that doesn't mean you can eat endless amounts without gaining weight. It still contains calories.

Truthfully, labels are not always as clear as the ice cream/non-fat yogurt comparison. For example, I picked up a carton of low-fat frozen yogurt at the grocery store. It seemed like a very healthy choice. However, after reading the label, I discovered that although it had less fat, the low-fat frozen yogurt contained far more sugar than the ice cream. Does that make it bad for you? Not necessarily. There is no simple answer; you have to look at the whole picture. Are there health concerns that would make a difference in your selection? Are you avoiding sugar? Perhaps you have already consumed enough high-fat foods for the day and so the low-fat frozen yogurt would be the more sensible choice. Perhaps you haven't had a high-fat treat in a long time and you have been true to the *Erase Your Waist* program. Half a cup of quality real ice cream could be just the thing to satisfy a craving. There needs to be balance in your diet. Enjoy variety and a selection of nutrients from all the food groups. Practice reading labels. You will get better at it. It's up to you to select the best foods to buy and eat. Take charge!

A Not-So-Final Note from the Author

I struggled for a long time trying to think what my parting words for you should be. Too many thoughts ran through my mind. There was one point where I got so frustrated that I wanted to say, "Oh! Just go eat a doughnut!" Just kidding! It finally hit me while I was sitting at an airport waiting to catch a red-eye. The problem I was having was that I didn't want to let go of you. You see, I really do care and sincerely hope that you will continue to make the *Erase Your Waist* a program for life. The reality is that it is truly in your hands now.

I am comforted that you now have a good source of practical information to incorporate into your life. We enjoyed some tummy talk together. That core knowledge will be a good reference should you need a refresher. You have a workout plan that will help you achieve dynamite abs. Promise me that you at least give it a try. It works! Keep up with your nutritional needs. Accept your genetics and body type. That alone with my fashion tips will carry you a long way. Always love and respect yourself inside and out. Small positive changes every day will add up to winning results.

For even more great information on how to look and feel your best pick up a copy of my book, *Your Best Bust*. I'd also love to share with you other healthy lifestyle tips. Visit my

website at www.starglow.com. Feel free to send me an email with your thoughts or comments. Good luck and remember—when the day is done the act of self-empowerment is in your hands. When it comes to *Erase Your Waist, you* take charge!

About the Author

Cyndi Targosz is a nationally recognized lifestyle/fitness expert and a motivational speaker. She is certified by ACE, AFAA, and AALC. Her fitness video and audio programs have sold over a half million copies. A graduate of Wayne State University, Cyndi obtained her degree in speech pathology and anatomy and physiology.

Her background includes work as an actress, model, dancer, radio personality, voiceover artist, and singer. All of these experiences have factored as elements of Cyndi's core belief of enjoying and having passion in the journey while setting realistic goals. She has successfully exhibited this philosophy in her M.B.S. System™ (Mind, Body, Spirit), where the mind must be centered, the body must be cared for, and the spirit must be fed. As president and CEO of her own company, STARGLOW Productions, Inc., Cyndi's clientele have included Hollywood actors, actresses, models, athletes, and other celebrities. Her clientele have included such major firms as Pacific Bell, Kaiser Permanente, Royal Caribbean Cruises, and Volkswagen of America, and many others. Contribution of her time and talents have been felt by numerous charitable organizations, among them the American Cancer Society, the YWCA, and the Girl Scouts of America. She is a frequent guest expert on numerous radio and television shows. Cyndi's personal philosophy maintains a focus on the interrelationship of balance on the inner and outer glow that provides all encompassing health, beauty, and wellness. Visit www.STARGLOW.com for more information about Cyndi Targosz.